COUGH CURES

**THE COMPLETE GUIDE TO THE BEST NATURAL
REMEDIES AND OVER-THE-COUNTER DRUGS
FOR ACUTE AND CHRONIC COUGHS**

GUSTAVO FERRER, MD &
BURKE LENNIHAN, RN, CCH

❧ **Moxie Life Press** ❧

Photographs of Dr. Gustavo Ferrer, and of Nicole Ferrer on page 34: Jayson Escalona
Photograph of Burke Lennihan: Savas Studios
Photograph of romerillo: Forest and Kim Starr
Front cover design and illustrations: Let's Write Books, Inc.

ISBN (paper): 978-0-9973307-0-0
ISBN (ebook): 978-0-9973307-1-7
Library of Congress Control Number: 2016904677

Moxie Life Press, Weston, FL
www.coughcuresbook.com
Printed in the United States of America

❧ DEDICATION ❧

To the love of my life, Nicole, the inspiration for this book. You provide the best medicine to all you touch: Love.

To my beloved children, Diego, Amanda and Lauren. You are the highlight of my days. May you pass the knowledge from this book to the next generation. I am very proud of you all!

—Dr. Gus

To all the courageous physicians who are pioneers in bringing natural healing to the world of mainstream medicine.

—Burke Lennihan

❧ CONTENTS ❧

TABLES

SHORTCUT GUIDES

ILLUSTRATIONS

❧ PREFACE ❧

Health care in the U.S. is in crisis. Costs increasing by double dig-its every year are breaking the budgets of cities, states and the fed-eral government, while 50% of what would otherwise be corporate profits are being eaten up by employee healthcare costs. Brilliant experts have proposed solutions: Stephen Brill in *America's Bitter Pill* highlights huge charges even at nonprofit hospitals and proposes greater transparency plus integrated hospitals and insurance systems. Jonathan Bush, founder of athenahealth and author of *Where Does It Hurt?*, suggests bringing in "disruptive innovation" in the form of the latest cloud-based software for more efficient delivery of health care. Dr. Gilbert Welch in *Overdiagnosed* proposes fewer screening tests and interventions as a way to improve our health while lowering costs.

But what about the actual care being delivered? The "best" and most expensive health care in the world places the United States below all other industrialized nations, down among the developing nations, in many measures of public health. Nearly every other country in the world includes some form of holistic health care—whether herbal medicine, homeopathy or Traditional Chinese Medicine—as part of its mainstream health care system, in the process saving money and ensuring better overall health for its citizens. In France—with the best health care in the world, according to the World Health Organiza-tion—95% of general practitioners and pediatricians prescribe homeo-pathic remedies, usually as part of a conventional medical practice.

i

Cuba has notably achieved health outcomes comparable to ours at only 4% of the cost. That's right—longevity and other parameters similar to the United States' for only 1/25th of the cost. How did they do it? To be sure, Cuba's hospitals are shabby and dilapidated for lack of funds. One positive factor, though: faced with a shortage of drugs due to the embargo, Cuba developed its "green medicine" based on herbal and homeopathic medicines.

It is no coincidence that Dr. Ferrer is Cuban, scion of the green medicine tradition, as we propose a healthcare innovation as old as the hills and as new as the latest research in physics. This book is an attempt to bridge the chasm that now separates natural-health-seeking patients from physicians who prescribe pharmaceuticals. Every time patients use an inexpensive natural medicine that works, they are saving money for themselves and for the whole health care system—but research shows that they are not telling their doctors!

The change we propose is already happening in America. Consumers are taking matters into their own hands, searching the internet for natural solutions, finding herbs and remedies that work better than their prescribed drugs.

Meanwhile physicians are also quietly consulting holistic practitioners for their own health problems, as Burke Lennihan can attest, having faculty from Harvard Medical School and physicians from the Harvard teaching hospitals as clients in her homeopathy practice.

We present here practical information about treating coughs, for the patient and busy doctor alike, while summarizing more than 200 research studies to validate our recommendations. Especially hoping to welcome physicians, hospital administrators and insurance executives into the conversation, we have attempted to convey in this book the mutually respectful and appreciative relationship between the authors who created it.

The medical information in this book is the contribution of Dr. Gustavo Ferrer, who grew up in rural Cuba with his grandmother and her herbs acting as the village healer and pharmacy. He went to medical school in Cuba, where he discovered his professors secretly going home to their herbalist grandmothers when they became ill. Redoing his internship and residency after coming to this country, Dr. Gus has become a pulmonologist who uses herbal and homeopathic medicines in his own home and recommends them to his patients.

The information about natural medicines herein is from Burke Lennihan, who went to Harvard expecting to become a physician like her father but discovered natural healing instead. She then operated a health food store where she learned about herbal medicine (the "old as the hills" part of our proposal) and now practices as a homeopath (the "new as the latest research in physics" part).

Burke also credits conventional medicine with saving her life during a health crisis ten years ago. So we have two authors, each an expert in one aspect of the health care equation while rooted in and respecting the other aspect. From our own collaboration we hope to promote a positive and fruitful conversation, drawing on the best of both forms of health care to benefit our patients. We hope you will enjoy the reading of this book as much as we have enjoyed the writing of it.

— *Gustavo Ferrer, MD*
Founder, The Cough Center at Cleveland Clinic Florida
President, Intensive Care Experts
Assistant Clinical Professor of Medicine, Nova Southeastern University
Weston, Florida

— *Burke Lennihan, RN, CCH*
Certified Classical Homeopath
The Lydian Center for Innovative Healthcare
Cambridge, Mass.

❧ ONE ❧

The Inspiration for This Book

"Wake up, time for school!" a sleepy and tired mom managed to screech out as she sat up in bed. Her fluffy pink slippers shuffled across the dark living room. "Wake up, sleepy heads!" she said as she turned on the lights in a shambolic room sprinkled with Barbies, Legos, ribbons, hair clips, and such. She checked up on Lauren, her five-year-old, who had been up half the night coughing despite the over-the-counter medication she had given her. She seemed fine. Then she made her way through the obstacle course to Amanda's bed, where her eight-year-old lay face down. She leaned over and gently caressed her back. She noticed that Amanda's body temperature was slightly higher than usual.

Mom ran off to get ready. A few minutes later she returned to the girls' room and to her surprise they were fast asleep. "No, no, no, get up! You have to go to school, you are going to be late!" Wishing her husband were home to relieve her, she called him, but there was no answer. He was gone from dusk to dawn working the night shift. She had no choice but to take care of things herself.

Amanda's fever was concerning, so Mom dashed to the medicine cabinet. She found some Mucinex and because she was pressed for time decided to give it to Amanda, even though it contained a decongestant and antihistamine for symptoms that her daughter didn't have. But the medication had expired—thank goodness she noticed before giving it to Amanda. She quickly

I

double-checked her fever with the Cuban method: a kiss on her daughter's forehead to feel her temperature. Sure enough, her fever was pretty high. She decided to keep Amanda home and take Lauren to school. Amanda did not have much of an appetite and left half her breakfast on her plate, but Lauren ate everything and downed it fast. Once in the car, when Lauren complained of a tummy ache, Mom explained that it was probably because she ate too fast.

She dropped Lauren off at school, late of course. To add to her distress, it started to pour. Amanda was in the back seat with glazed-over, half-closed eyes. She told her mom that her throat hurt. So it was off to the drug store for fever and sore throat medications.

Amanda was underage so of course Mom had to bring her in. Struggling with the umbrella, she managed to keep Amanda dry while she herself got drenched.

Standing in front of what seemed to be a 100-foot wall with every medication available, she thought, "Which one do I choose?" Suddenly her cellphone rang. The call was from the school — Lauren was suffering from diarrhea and she needed to be picked up. Exhausted from a sleepless night, soaking wet and now rushed, Mom had to quickly select the correct medicines to provide her children with the best treatment for their symptoms.

The exhausted, confused and busy Mom in this situation is my wife. After she told me her story, I was determined to teach her all I know about coughs and colds and how to choose the most appropriate treatments when I am not home. She is the inspiration that gave birth to this book. Here is what I told her.

Many times a cold begins with a tickle at the back of the throat or a sore throat closely followed by a stuffy and/or runny nose followed by a cough. Sometimes headaches, fever, and sinus pressure can develop. People who visit the doctor for these symptoms will receive a prescription for some sort of symptomatic relief. But symptoms tend to keep changing as part of the natural progression of a viral infection, so a prescription that works one day may not be effective by the following day.

Therefore, in desperation (and trusting the pharmacy never sells anything that's not good for you) patients turn to an over-the-counter drug, favoring one (maybe unconsciously) they recognize from a television commercial. They choose medications based on the description on the front, without examining the active ingredients. And with the lengthy names that only health care professionals recognize, how can the average person know or understand the fine print? They often end up choosing a combination medication that contains more drugs than they need.

To make matters worse, most health care professionals don't understand that there are only minor differences between the common cold, an acute cough, flu-like illness and flu itself. All of them are about the same with the exception of complicated flu, where symptoms are more severe and pneumonia is a common complication. The lingo is confusing and misused. For instance, after you have a week of a nagging cough, stuffy and runny nose, low-grade fever, fatigue, achy muscles, and sinus pressure, one doctor may diagnose bronchitis and another may label it a common cold.

While writing this book, I conducted a survey of more than 200 female patients, their ages ranging from 20 to 90 and with varying educational backgrounds. They used herbal remedies, teas, menthol inhalations, and homeopathic medicines to treat colds and coughs. Not considering them drugs, they failed to report them during a doctor visit. The practitioner unaware of these remedies may prescribe medications whose effect is blocked or enhanced by them, a situation called "drug-drug interaction." (And yes, herbs can interact with drugs just as other drugs can).

Healthcare professionals often lack training in how to treat acute coughs and common colds, leaving the doors wide open for patients to choose their own over-the-counter treatments in a market dominated by advertising. This is made worse by the confusion ignited by media and advertising and further distorted by misinformation on the Internet.

The best of both worlds

I am in the fortunate position of being a fully trained conventional doctor who grew up using herbal teas and folk remedies extensively for coughs and colds. In this book I want to share with you the best of both of these worlds. But first, let me tell you my story.

I grew up in the eastern mountains of Cuba, from a long line of farmers who grow the most delicious, succulent mangos in the world. In my hometown with a population of less than a thousand, we learned to depend on homemade remedies such as teas, herbal plasters and many other natural concoctions to treat illnesses such as acute cough, common cold, nausea, vomiting and indigestion. We only visited the doctor in dire emergencies. For everything else, it was grandma to the rescue. And rest assured, she had a homemade remedy for just about anything.

It wasn't until 1981 that the first doctor's office was opened in Palmar, my hometown. Prior to that, going to the doctor was an agonizing whole-day ordeal. For our annual physical, my mom would wake us up at 5 am, without breakfast of course, because we were about to have blood work done. Without a vehicle at our disposal, most families traveled by tractor-trailer, truck or whatever else was going our way. The distance to the doctor's office was only about 16 miles, but countless times it took us the entire day. Conditions were tough and not much was available to doctors — only a few injectable pain medications, some syringes, bottles of saline, blood pressure medications and the occasional antibiotics. Therefore, doctors as well as families turned to home remedies to treat common diseases.

Years later, my dad managed to buy an antiquated 1955 jeep that became our town's ambulance. It was in the back of this jeep, one moonlit night when I was 15, that I discovered my life mission to be a doctor. I had spotted a pregnant woman walking down from the hills, barefoot and exhausted, feebly begging for help. I alerted my dad, and as he raced the dilapidated jeep over the potholes on the way to the hospital, I climbed into the back seat to help her give birth, following my dad's shouted orders. As I caught the baby girl, I witnessed the miracle of life unfolding before me and saw her take her first breath of life. From that day on I knew I wanted to be a doctor.

The breath of life always captivated me, so when I went to medical school I became a pulmonologist treating respiratory illnesses. My pulmonary education in Cuba consisted of 100 percent Western medicine. (This was a few years before the Cuban government decided to focus on developing its "green medicine," anticipating a shortage of drugs due to the embargo.) We were trained to only use pharmaceutical medications approved in America and Europe. Our professors discouraged any use of home remedies, claiming they lacked scientific evidence. However, I found myself, the "westernized" pulmonologist, calling grandma when I had a cold. In fact, later on I found out that my professors too, called their moms or grandmas when they were sick. Obviously, Western medicine did not convince them enough for them to use it themselves!

After I had completed my medical training, I led a United Nations research project searching for tuberculosis among the native Indians of Venezuela's Orinoco River basin. I found a common thread between the Venezuelan doctors and my Cuban colleagues: they were trained in Western medicine, yet relied more on natural remedies.

Tired of the lack of freedom my country offered and wanting to expand my horizons, I set my compass north to America, the land of opportunities. Although I didn't speak an ounce of English, I was determined to learn the language. Within two years, I was able to enroll in a three-year residency at Texas Tech University followed by a three-year fellowship in pulmonary and critical care at George Washington University. Yes! I had to do internal medicine and pulmonary training all over again. My wife likes to call me Dr. Squared!

Remember what's important to the patient

Although it was a difficult journey, I have never regretted it for one moment. It was in those years that I learned to look at medicine from my patients' perspective. During these years of training I had the privilege of meeting physicians, nurses and healthcare professionals from every corner of the world. Always curious, I would inquire as to how they practiced medicine in their countries and how it compared to American medicine. Invariably, our conversations evolved around the availability of medications, cancer treatments, or advanced cardiovascular procedures. We seldom talked about commonplace issues such as smoking, diet, exercise, back pain, headaches, common colds, acute coughs and flus.

Every year I participate in the world's most prestigious meetings in pulmonary medicine (the conferences of the American Thoracic Society and American College of Chest Physicians), where thousands of research projects are presented and discussed. And again, I find that the common cold, acute cough illness and flu are seldom part of the discussion. In fact, out of a thousand studies discussed at the American Thoracic Society in 2012, only three were on chronic coughs and none on acute coughs and colds. It seems that these are not significant enough for medical professionals.

However, a recent study entitled "Why Patients Visit their Doctors" conducted by the Mayo Clinic says otherwise.* The Mayo study found that coughs and colds were among the most prevalent complaint in all age groups. It concluded by recommending that research focus on the most common reasons for doctor visits — the exact opposite of the research priorities of the professional societies.

At this point, you might be thinking, "So what's the big deal? Don't we have over-the-counter drugs to treat coughs and colds? No one has died, right? Well, my dear friends, acetaminophen, often sold as Tylenol, is the most common cause of liver failure worldwide and therefore yes, people have died from it.**

---

*See the Endnotes for research studies to support statements like this in the text. Research studies documenting the effectiveness of herbal medicines are collated for convenience in Appendix D, of homeopathic medicines in Appendix E, and of natural therapies in Appendix F.

**Tylenol is the common name for acetaminophen. I have chosen to use both names in most instances when the drug is mentioned in this book because most people know it as Tylenol, but they need to recognize "acetaminophen" on the medication label.

A cautionary note about Tylenol

Acetaminophen shows up in so many different cold remedies, pain medications and sleeping pills that people don't realize they can easily exceed the safe daily limit. Most people have trouble reading the labels, and it is it is unfortunately easy to take too much of a medication with significant toxicity that can cost you your health or worse, your life. Most liver failures ending up in transplant are due to the unintentional ingestion of acetaminophen/Tylenol.

Carol,* a 52-year-old business executive, was brought to me in the Intensive Care Unit (ICU) vomiting blood. She had been diagnosed with fibromyalgia the previous year because she had significant pain in all her muscles. Six months earlier, her doctor had advised her to exercise. Although she tried to improve her health by walking three times a week, the pain was unbearable, so—following the instructions on the label—she would take a couple of extra strength acetaminophen/ Tylenol (500 mg each) every six to eight hours. Because the pain interrupted her sleep, she also started taking Tylenol PM, which is a combination of 500 mg of acetaminophen and 25 mg of diphenhydramine (Benadryl).

About a week or so prior to her arrival at the ICU, she developed a stuffy nose, sore throat and runny nose. She went to the pharmacy and purchased a cold remedy that read, "Sore throat, cough, sneezing and stuffy nose." She wasn't aware that the medicine contained another 500 mg of acetaminophen/Tylenol combined with a decongestant, an antihistamine, and a cough suppressant. She took this medicine every 8 hours, following the instructions on the label, along with the acetaminophen/Tylenol for her pain and Tylenol PM to sleep.

After three days the sore throat subsided. However, now her symptoms evolved into a persistent cough and a stuffy, runny nose.

---

*Names and identifying characteristics of patients have been changed to protect their privacy, however the details of their condition and their care are all authentic.

Off to the pharmacy she went. Confused by her symptoms, she asked the pharmacist for advice. "I like hot teas when I'm sick, so why don't you try the Theraflu tea?" he said. Carol remembered her own mother giving her a soothing herbal tea when she was sick and this made the choice appealing. The cough and cold aisle offered nine choices of Theraflu. The word "Max" in Theraflu Max-D allured her. She did not realize that this too contained a whopping 1000 mg of acetaminophen/Tylenol combined with an antihistamine and a decongestant.

Shortly after adding "Max" to the mix she began vomiting blood and was rushed to the hospital. After a blood transfusion in the emergency room she was transferred to me at the ICU. Upon carefully reviewing her history carefully, I told her that she had ruptured a vein in her esophagus. Shocked, she replied, "How could this happen? I don't drink alcohol. Isn't this what happens to alcoholics?"

I told her it was due to liver failure and the most likely cause was an acetaminophen overdose. "I didn't try to kill myself," she replied, quite upset. I mentioned that unintentional acetaminophen/Tylenol overdose was the most common cause of liver failure in America. She couldn't believe it, so to prove it we added up the doses of acetaminophen in the pills she had ingested over a 24 hour period.

Extra Strength Tylenol: two 500 mg every 8 hours	3,000 mg
Tylenol PM: 500 mg at bed time	500 mg
Sudafed Cough/Cold: 500 mg every 8 hours	1,500 mg
Theraflu Max-D: 1000 mg every 8 hours	3,000 mg
Daily Total	**8,000 mg**

The FDA recently reduced the safe upper limit for a daily dose of acetaminophen from 4000 mg to 3000 mg. She had just taken nearly three times the safe upper limit without even realizing it!

Fortunately, the bleeding subsided while she was in the ICU without a doctor's intervention. I told her to discontinue all the combination medications that contained acetaminophen/Tylenol. I taught her my system of alternatives for the treatment of coughs, colds and pain: a combination of natural teas, homeopathic medicines and acupressure. For her chronic pain, I recommended massages, relaxation, breathing exercises, acupuncture and supplements. I also taught her how to read the labels on over-the-counter medications and to choose them carefully. Thankfully, her life was transformed in a matter of months and her liver was healed. Not all patients suffering from an acetaminophen overdose are so lucky.

Informative solutions and healthy blessings

How can we resolve this dilemma? The solution is at hand. As Nelson Mandela said, "Education is the most powerful weapon we can use to change the world." Let's use this power. My intention is not to create a new dogmatic system but to inform. Like C.S. Lewis, I do not want "to cut down jungles but to irrigate deserts."

In this book I will teach you the principles I've shared with my wife and my patients. I will give you a simple and clear understanding of how to treat coughs and colds by combining herbs, homeopathic medicines, acupressure, supplements, breathing exercises, meditation, prayer, and many other well-researched alternatives.

Whether you prefer over-the-counter medications or the natural approach, this book will help you to confidently navigate the options, choose an appropriate treatment for your symptoms, and avoid a potentially dangerous combination of medications. You will save time and money as well as securing a healthier life.

Are You Taking Too Much Tylenol?

Gather the bottles of medications you take on a daily basis and write down the following for each medicine that contains acetaminophen:

ॐ the amount of acetaminophen in each tablet (mgs)

ॐ the number of tablets you take for each dose

ॐ the number of doses you take in a day.

Multiply the amount of acetaminophen by the number of tablets and then by the number of doses. Repeat for each medication that you are on. Finally, add up the total for each day.

Medication	Mgs	Pills Per Dose	Doses Per Day	Total
_____	_____	X _____	X _____	= _____
_____	_____	X _____	X _____	= _____
_____	_____	X _____	X _____	= _____
_____	_____	X _____	X _____	= _____
_____	_____	X _____	X _____	= _____
_____	_____	X _____	X _____	= _____
_____	_____	X _____	X _____	= _____

TOTAL PER DAY= _____

How does it compare to the FDA's 3000 mg safe upper limit? Are you taking less? Well done!

I recommend only 1500 mg as a safe upper limit, because I observed people still rushing to the emergency room with symptoms of acetaminophen poisoning after the FDA lowered the limit from 6000 mg to 3000 mg a day.

TWO

To Google or Not to Google?

Cathy, a 50-year-old journalist, came to my cough clinic with a per-sistent dry cough. Ignoring the receptionist's friendly greeting, she created a little mobile office in the waiting room, spreading out her iPad and files on the neighboring chairs. Her cellphone rang like a fire alarm, but before she could answer it, she had a coughing fit that left her speechless. Soon after, Esther the nurse — another friendly face—called her in to see me, but Cathy didn't acknowl-edge her smile either. Frustrated, she stormed past Esther, who asked, "How long have you had this cough?"

"Months!" Cathy barked. "This cough is driving me crazy, and it's interfering with my job because I can't interview my sources. My boss told me I need to take care of this cough—or else."

"I understand," Esther replied.

"How can you possibly understand? You're not the one cough-ing," Cathy replied with tear-filled eyes.

"You're right. I don't have a cough, but we help people here every day. I'm sure we can do the same for you. Dr. Gus wants to help everyone with coughs. He's even writing a book about coughs."

"A book on coughs? Who needs a book about coughs? I just go to the pharmacy or online and get all the information I need," Cathy replied.

"If that were true, maybe you wouldn't be here," Esther responded kindly. "Dr. Gus says that pharmacists often recommend cough

medicines which they know don't work and can cause side effects, because they have nothing better to offer. They haven't been trained in the natural medicines right in their own pharmacy. And going to the Internet for answers can steer you the wrong way."

We see people as frustrated as Cathy in our clinic every day, frustrated by the cough that is keeping them awake and maybe costing them their jobs. They are also frustrated because they've gone from doctor to doctor without relief. By the time patients come to a specialized clinic like ours, some of them have been to ten different doctors. They come in to our clinic frustrated with us in advance because they expect to get yet another medication which does not work.

My heart goes out to patients like Cathy. I appreciate their frustration. I also sympathize with my fellow physicians who have not been taught effective ways to treat coughs. I have been blessed with the ability to solve these difficult cough cases, because I take the time to really listen before recommending an individualized integrative treatment plan. When I first interview a patient, I do not take notes, I do not use a computer, I just listen sympathetically and respectfully until we uncover the reason underlying the cough.

Cathy calmed down right away when she realized I was really listening to her. It turned out that stress at work was a trigger for her cough. With circulation declining at her newspaper, staff was being cut, and now her editor was threatening to use her cough as an excuse to cut her job as well. The stress made her turn to emotional eating of lots of junk food.

I explained to her that she needed to clean up her diet and eat healthier food. I taught her some breathing exercises to calm her cough and her anxiety. I also recommended some supplements and a homeopathic remedy for people who are anxious about survival issues: work, money, and health. Three months later at her followup visit her cough was gone, her mood was much better, and she was interviewing for a job at a larger newspaper.

The Internet and the art of medicine

Now back to Cathy's confidence in the Internet as a source of information. Unfortunately, this is a critical problem in today's society. Cathy is a journalist whose profession depends on sourcing accurate information, but she was unaware that the Internet can be an extremely unreliable or misleading source of medical information.

Yes, there are reliable websites like WebMD.com, MayoClinic.org, and ClevelandClinic.org, but some patients use them in a way that interferes with their care. Patients arrive at a doctor's appointment these days with a sheaf of papers printed out from the Internet and their minds already made up as to their diagnosis. They have already decided the medication they need based on an ad they saw on TV.

This means that doctors cannot explore the patient's symptoms with an unbiased mind and determine the best treatment from a wider range of options than patients are aware of. The doctor's thinking is stifled and the patient does not tell the whole story, because she has already decided which symptoms are related to her predetermined diagnosis.

But medicine is an art that uses scientific data to correct or improve medical problems in the canvas of life. This art cannot be found on the internet (I explain in Chapter 11). The patient's emotions are at the heart of this concept. The art of medicine is multifaceted and includes deeply listening to the patient; interacting with sensitivity, compassion and support; discovering the underlying emotional stresses; using a holistic approach; and making lifestyle recommendations.

Internet information interferes in another way: filling the patient's mind with anxiety about imagined illnesses. Typically from the time a primary care physician refers a patient to a pulmonologist (lung specialist) like me, it takes three months to get an appointment. Let's say a CAT scan shows a nodule (small growth) on the lung. CAT scans are so powerful now, the "false positives" are skyrocketing. These are indistinct blurs on the image that seem to indicate a disease and require a referral to a specialist, but turn out to be nothing.

During the three months that patients wait to see me, typically they go on the Internet to see what a nodule on the lung might mean. They become convinced they have cancer or fibrosis of the lung, they become anxious and they can't sleep. One of the symptoms we lung specialists use for a diagnosis is shortness of breath. But anxiety can *cause* shortness of breath!

Patients will tell me, "I have a nodule on my lung," and I say, "I have a nodule on my lung too! They are common and most of the time they don't mean anything." I run some more tests and in the great majority of cases I am able to tell the patient that she is fine. (I am careful to say that she is healthy as of that day and we cannot tell what the future will bring.) Meanwhile she has spent three months scouring the Internet, believing she has cancer. It's like a survival mechanism in a primitive part of the brain: people focus on the worst possible outcome. I have to spend a lot of time with these patients educating them and reassuring them.

Beware of herbs from the internet

Another huge problem I see with the Internet: people search for information about natural healing, and some of the top websites that come up are those of hackers and scammers. These websites prey on people in pain, getting their credit card information by claiming magic results for purported herbal remedies. People come to my clinic with herbal remedies from China and other countries; these herbs and supplements are entirely unregulated and may have no active ingredients or may even have toxins.

The most reliable supplements sold in the U.S. come from reputable companies with clean sources of supply. Be especially wary of herbs from China where heavy metals have contaminated the soil. Even supplements bottled in the U.S. may use polluted herbs from China or poor quality herbs from other countries. We recommend Gaia Herbs because the company grows its own organic herbs here in the U.S. and tests the plants for the active ingredients. Herb Pharm, Planetary Formulas and Solaray are other reliable sources.

But developing countries have no regulations for herb and supplement manufacture, and my Hispanic patients are especially vulnerable. The Spanish-language websites feature herbs of unknown medicinal value from around the world, and I see my Hispanic patients frequently falling prey to the allure of their claims.

As for asking a pharmacist for information, when you ask a question at the pharmacy counter, you are most likely talking to pharmacy techs who are not trained in over-the-counter medications. The professional pharmacists are busy in the back and only talk to customers on request.

Avoiding unnecessary antibiotics for coughs, colds and flu

Why a book about coughs in particular? Among Google searches on health topics in 2015, three of the top ten were about coughs. Coughs and colds are one of the most common reasons for doctor visits and for missed workdays/school days in the US, yet doctors are not properly trained in treating upper respiratory infections. Most over-the-counter drugs for coughs and colds are ineffective at best, harmful at worst. The pharmaceutical industry, focused on chronic diseases and the major causes of death, has neglected these everyday infections that result in 100 million physician visits a year.

Sadly, two-thirds of patients with coughs are prescribed unnecessary antibiotics on their first visit. Most acute coughs are caused by colds and flu, which are viral, and antibiotics do not work for viral infections. Lacking effective drugs for viral infections, physicians can only recommend fluids and bed rest. But they are pressured by their patients to prescribe *something*, so doctors tend to prescribe antibiotics. Because they do not work, patients get stronger antibiotics on subsequent visits, which means that chronic cough sufferers tend to be way overmedicated with antibiotics.

These unnecessary antibiotics add to the cost of health care and can cause side effects ranging from the annoying to the serious. Studies show that antibiotics can affect the kidneys (even causing kidney failure), vision (retinal detachment), muscles and tendons (tendon rupture), the central nervous system (brain fog), and the digestive system (diarrhea). They reduce overall energy levels by attacking the mitochondria, the powerhouses of the cell.

This overuse of antibiotics contributes to the development of antibiotic-resistant bacteria. Bacteria are smart. Multiplying at a formidable rate, they can mutate so that they are resistant to a particular antibiotic. Once one strain develops resistance, it can quickly pass this "secret weapon" along to other types of bacteria in little packets of information called plasmids. Gradually that antibiotic loses effectiveness against a wide swath of disease-causing bugs. Meanwhile it takes years to develop a new antibiotic and put it through all the required testing. At this point in time there are few antibiotics under development for antibiotic-resistant bacteria. The World Health Organization calls antibiotic resistance "a problem so serious that it threatens the achievements of modern medicine. A post-antibiotic era, in which common infections and minor injuries can kill, far from being an apocalyptic fantasy, is instead a very real possibility for the 21st century." In the US, the FDA and CDC have asked physicians to stop prescribing antibiotics, and in 2015 a National Action Plan was created to reduce their use.

Concerns with other over-the-counter drugs

We need safe and effective alternatives to prescription antibiotics. What about over-the-counter (OTC) drugs? Americans spend $40 billion annually on OTC drugs, many of which provide little, if any, symptomatic relief. And some are potentially so toxic that many people actually put their lives in danger with common OTC medications. New evidence indicates that Tylenol (acetaminophen) blocks the mitochondria (energy-producing elements in cells); increases the risk of asthma; and depletes glutathione. Losing glutathione affects our health in many ways, because it is the master antioxidant, essential for our immune system, for longevity and for getting rid of the toxins so prevalent in our world.

A recent survey of thousands of consumers found that:

- ∿ Consumers believe that OTC medications are extremely safe and not likely to lead to serious toxicity.

∾ Most consumers do not read labels on medications.

∾ Some medications are not adequately labeled.

∾ Consumers are not aware that potentially harmful acetamino-phen is hidden in most OTC combination medications for coughs, colds and flu.

The danger of liver failure from taking just a handful of common OTC drugs has become such a problem that the Acute Liver Failure Study Group has recommended eliminating all OTC drugs in which acetaminophen is combined with other drugs. The group has tried unsuccessfully for more than 10 years now to ban these combination products because it's too easy to get an accidental overdose from them.

Even if cough medications do not contain acetaminophen, they can still cause problems. The American Academy of Pediatrics stressed in a 2008 public health advisory that "over-the-counter cough and cold medicines do not work for children younger than 6 years of age and in some cases may pose a significant health risk." It advised against giving cough or cold medications to children 2 and under "because of serious and life-threatening side effects."

Not all cough medications are harmful, of course. But do they work? One of the nation's leading experts on coughs — Dr. Richard Irwin, chairman of the cough guidelines committee of the American College of Chest Physicians and editor of the journal *CHEST* — has stated: "OTCs contain combinations of drugs that have *never been proven to treat coughs.*" [italics added] The European Respiratory Society and the Canadian Respiratory Society have a similar position when it comes to OTC drugs for coughs.

Patients are discovering natural remedies on their own

So my fellow physicians are left with ineffective or even harmful medi-cines to prescribe or recommend to patients. Meanwhile, whether we know it or not, many of our patients are exploring natural treatments on their own, and the number is increasing each year. The landmark 1993 study that first documented Americans going to holistic practitioners more often than to their primary care doctors also revealed that the great majority never shared that information with their doctors. Many of these traditional remedies have had their usefulness validated by scientific research, but these studies are not included in the curriculum of medical schools. They have not crossed the great chasm in our society that divides conventional medicine from natural healing. My colleagues do not feel comfortable recommending natural strategies that they consider "unproven," unaware of the many research studies that support their use.

To add to the confusion, the Internet (what I like to call the "world wild web") is filled with lots of false information about medical issues. With thousands, even millions of people posting their opinions and their experiences regarding natural treatments, it can be difficult to know what to believe. Sadly, I see in my practice every day how confused my patients have become from the conflicting information on the web. I tell them the web can be like the Tower of Babel: confusing and divisive.

Adding even more to the confusion, most physicians are just not properly trained in how to diagnose and treat acute coughs *because that is not part of the curriculum in most medical schools worldwide.* These curriculums focus on chronic illnesses and the latest high-power drugs developed to treat them, because medical students want to go into a specialty rather than into family practice. We desperately need a reliable system to treat coughs, one that does not over-promise and under-deliver, while providing the best available treatment options and opening the doors to more worthwhile research. This book starts the dialog to create that system.

Let's start with answers to my patients' most common questions.

Are all OTC medications approved by the FDA?

The approval process for OTC medications is much simpler than for prescription drugs, which require years of trials costing hundreds of millions of dollars. With more than 300,000 OTC drug products on the market, the FDA can do little more than review the ingredients and labeling of each one.

The ingredients in many OTC medications are made from drugs that were formerly "by prescription only" and therefore have gone through a strict approval process (but it also means they may not really be safe enough to take without a physician's oversight). When these drugs went off patent, the manufacturer typically applied for permission to sell them over the counter without a prescription, which would make it easier for consumers to buy them.

If OTC medications are *not* made from former prescription drugs, they must be made from *ingredients* approved by the FDA for each category of drug, like antacids, analgesics, and so forth.

Do supplements and herbs go through the FDA's "security check" too?
The security check for these products is more passive: manufacturers must inform the FDA that they will be marketing a new product and that they have research documenting its safety and efficacy, however they do not need to submit the research unless the FDA requests it. The FDA usually does not request it unless there are complaints about the product, although it occasionally makes periodic reviews of a particular category. The FDA does not test supplements, just as it does not test OTC drugs.

From the FDA website: "FDA regulates both finished dietary supplement products and dietary ingredients ... Manufacturers and distributors ... are prohibited from marketing products that are adulterated or misbranded. That means that these firms are responsible for evaluating the safety and labeling of their products before marketing to ensure that they meet all the requirements of DSHEA and FDA regulations. FDA is responsible for taking action against any adulterated or misbranded dietary supplement product after it reaches the market."

In addition the Federal Trade Commission (FTC) regulates claims about dietary supplements: companies may not claim that a dietary supplement can cure a disease or other health condition. However, they can claim that it addresses a nutrient deficiency, promotes good health, or supports bodily functions indicated on the label. Also, the label should include a disclaimer stating that it has not been evaluated by the FDA.

On many vitamin labels, you can see the FDA's recommended wording, "These statements have not been evaluated by the Food and Drug Administration. This product is not intended to diagnose, treat, cure or prevent any disease." This does not mean that the product does not work; in the case of Vitamins C and D, for example, there are hundreds if not thousands of research studies. It simply means the FDA has not evaluated them.

As for supplement manufacturers following Good Manufacturing Processes, you can generally trust supplements sold in stores and through health care practitioners, but beware of ones sold only on the Internet.

Does homeopathic medicine work?

Absolutely! I can say this from my own experience, because my family and I have had excellent results with cough-specific homeopathic treatments. In fact, I just bought a homeopathic cough syrup for one of my daughters, and her cough was gone in a couple of days, faster than I would have expected. I suggest homeopathic treatments to my patients, who have also had excellent results. Homeopathy is a system of natural medicine using highly diluted and energized medicinal substances, given mainly in tablet form, to trigger the body's natural system of healing. The remedies store information, somewhat like a flash drive or CD disk, which they convey to the body's healing energy as explained in Chapter 6.

Homeopathy has gone down a rocky road of acceptance for more than 100 years in the US. While it is widely accepted in Europe, India, Russia, Canada and South America, it is widely considered "unproven" in the US because doctors are not familiar with the research studies. However, in recent times, the number of well-designed studies evaluating homeopathic remedies for specific conditions has increased substantially, and the research shows that for many symptoms and conditions such as upper respiratory infections the appropriate homeopathic remedies do indeed work. (See Appendix E for research on homeopathy.)

The latest research comparing a homeopathic cough syrup *alone* to the same cough syrup *plus* an antibiotic showed that not only did the homeopathic medicine work well, the antibiotic added no benefit — only side effects. In other words, cough sufferers would be better off with the homeopathic and no antibiotics. No press releases were issued for this study. No media outlets covered it. That's why you need this book!

Many of these products are well-known in Europe, however. For example, Oscillococcinum (or "Oscillo") is the most popular flu remedy in France. Its bright orange box is showing up in drugstores all over America. I have personally used Oscillococcinum for my children with excellent results. Overall, homeopathic medicines are harmless, free of side effects and tasteless — which is a plus for my children. No one likes to chase their kids around the house with a spoonful of yucky-tasting medication!

Grandma's remedies — do they work?

Yes, absolutely. Research has validated the effectiveness of many home-made remedies. We'll be describing them and their research in upcoming chapters. Grandma's remedies fell out of favor during the last hundred years with the discovery of antibiotics and other "miracle drugs." Now that we're finding the limitations of these drugs, we're realizing Grandma knew what she was doing. In the microcosm of your home and mine, these traditional remedies are often used and widely accepted, and I suspect you have experienced the healing effect of a nice hot bowl of homemade chicken soup. Since every culture, country, and region has developed its own homemade remedy formulas, the spectrum is vast and wide.

Of course not all homemade remedies are effective, and we'll advise you against several ineffective and potentially harmful homemade remedies and practices. You will learn how to create your own natural remedies using simple products from your kitchen cabinet or the health food store.

I'm way too busy to read a book on coughs.

Perhaps you are one of those extremely busy parents who opens her eyes to the sound of the annoying alarm in the morning, only to smack the snooze button several times before you finally get out of bed. You two-step it to your kids' room to wake them up, but they toss and turn in bed for a while before they too finally get up. A quick breakfast, then you shove the kids in the car and rush them to school. On your way, you go over their homework and plan the pick-up, all the while praying that the route is cop-free. "I can't afford another speeding ticket" is looping through your brain.

You drop the kids at school and it's off to a busy workday. Before you know it, it's three o'clock and you're back to the cycle until you collapse in bed at night. If this is you, you can't afford NOT to read this book—you can't afford to have you or your family members out sick. Also you are more likely to make a careless mistake and pick the wrong medication if you're in a rush.

On the other hand, if your life is extremely organized and balanced, that's wonderful. This book is for you too. It will help you become an expert at preventing and treating the cough associated with common colds, sinus problems and flu, and shortening the duration of symptoms, too.

Can't I just ask the pharmacist for help?

The pharmacist? Probably not. As we've explained before, pharmacists are busy behind the counter and rarely talk to customers, so you will probably get a pharmacy tech who is not trained to answer questions. Also they are not aware of the natural medicines now available in the nationwide pharmacy chains. I hope that this book will be useful in training pharmacy staff in the options they can offer their customers.

In the next chapter, we'll explore the medical lingo. However, if you have a nagging cough right now, please jump ahead to Appendix A for some immediate assistance. You can come back to this part later for the deeper knowledge that will help you take control of your health.

Doctor Alert:
When to See Your Doctor

Seek help if the cough is accompanied by any of the following:

- ∽ a fever lasting more than three days,
  even a low grade fever (100°/101°),
- ∽ chills with shaking,
- ∽ coughing up a large amount of phlegm
  (whitish, yellow or even green),
- ∽ coughing up blood or blood-streaked mucus,
- ∽ wheezing or significant shortness of breath,
- ∽ difficulty breathing or rapid breathing,
- ∽ chest pain with the cough or a deep breath,
- ∽ a rapid heartbeat (tachycardia), and/or
- ∽ lethargy/uncharacteristic drowsiness,
  especially in an infant or child.

A persistent cough with one or more of these symptoms, whether or not there is a lot of mucus, could mean pneumonia or bronchitis. You should immediately consult your doctor or visit the nearest urgent care or hospital emergency department.

Pneumonia (especially in an infant) is not always accompanied by a cough. Always seek medical help if your child has a fever, is breathing rapidly, and is limp and pale or otherwise seems unwell.

A cough lasting more than four to six weeks and showing no signs of improving on its own, especially if it is disrupting your sleep, needs investigating by a medical professional.

❧ THREE ❧

I Have *What?*
Understanding the Lingo

Elizabeth, 10-year-old Piper's mother, received a worried call from the school nurse: Piper was "coming down" with something, and she had chills, a sore throat and a persistent cough. Piper was waiting at the principal's office and greeted her mother with a frustrated look. "I don't want to miss dance class."

"Don't worry. We'll stop by the doctor's on the way home and tomorrow you'll be OK," she replied, but suddenly Piper had a coughing fit. Her eyes got watery and her nose stuffed up instantly, making it hard to breathe. Elizabeth scrambled through her purse, pulled out her iPhone and asked Siri for the closest pediatric urgent care center.

After a basic history and physical exam—including a look into the ears—the pediatrician said, "Don't worry, she only has a URI."

"A URI? What's that?" Elizabeth was both confused and embarrassed at her own ignorance.

"URI stands for upper respiratory infection, or really, just a common cold. They're the same. She probably has a cough caused by postnasal drip. Give her plenty of fluids and use acetaminophen for the fever up to three times a day. If she still has a fever after three days, call us or come back."

"How about for the cough?" Elizabeth asked.

"Oh, well, you can use over-the-counter Robitussin," the doctor

replied as he left the room.

That night the whole family didn't sleep a wink because of Piper's nonstop cough. She did not go to school the next day, and Elizabeth, worried, stayed home from work in order to take care of her. The Robitussin didn't help at all. By the third day, Piper's cough had not improved. Elizabeth took her back to the urgent care clinic, where a different pediatrician diagnosed Piper with bronchitis. He prescribed antibiotics, nebulizers several times a day and a different cough suppressant.

After another three days passed with no improvement, Elizabeth was able to get an appointment with Piper's own pediatrician, Dr. Mark. He listened to the story, checked Piper's lungs with a stethoscope, and said, "It sounds like she might have asthma. I'm going to refer you to a specialist because it can be difficult for doctors like me to diagnose asthma at the very early stage."

"Asthma?" Elizabeth replied with surprise. "But Dr. Mark, she's never had asthma before. Asthma sounds really serious. Will the medication be harmful?"

"Don't worry," Dr. Mark replied. "It's probably just a cough, but I want to make sure. If she does have asthma, she can control it with an inhaler. The new inhalers use just a fraction of a fraction of the drugs that the older ones did. They are just as effective with a tiny amount of the medicine. I understand your concern, and not to worry!"

Elizabeth was surprised that her daughter had been given a possible diagnosis of five different medical conditions in just a few days (cough, upper respiratory infection, postnasal drip, bronchitis and asthma). Fortunately, the pulmonologist diagnosed Piper with postnasal drip. Elizabeth was not aware that our current healthcare system requires doctors to specify a diagnosis, and it's difficult to tell the difference among different types of coughs without specialized tests — tests we physicians only request if the obvious medications are not working. My colleagues sincerely try to do their best for their patients within the limited time of their appointments.

We usually don't see patients in my clinic who have only had one coughing fit like Piper's, because the wait is too long. Fortunately Elizabeth and Piper are our neighbors. When Elizabeth told me that she was still worried that Piper might have asthma, I reassured her that Dr. Mark was just trying to be extra cautious.

In fact asthma does not show up with cold symptoms. Cold symptoms are in the head (runny nose, sore throat, postnasal drip) while asthma symptoms are in the chest (narrowed airways and extra mucus causing shortness of breath and a wheeze when breathing out). I told Elizabeth about some herbs and homeopathics to have on hand for the next time Piper had a cold or coughing fit. I also encouraged her to call me if Piper's cough became a problem, but it's been almost a year now without any distress calls.

In this chapter we are going to dive into the terminology, symptoms and diseases that form the backbone of the entire book. Wait! Wait! Keep reading.

Before you skip these pages and jump headlong to the next chapter, give me a moment to explain what I have here for you. This section explains why and how we cough in plain English — English so simple that you won't even catch my Cuban accent. Illustrations will help you grasp the real essence. I use these illustrations in my clinic to easily explain medical problems for my patients. With a grasp of this section, you can understand your doctors and help give them the information they need. So bear with me while we dig into this very important section.

Why do we cough?

Coughing is an important defense mechanism. Yes, it serves many social functions, like interrupting an inappropriate conversation. Physically, coughing clears your airways of particles and secretions, and it protects you from breathing foreign materials into your lungs where they could cause an infection. It protects the lungs from dust, micro-organisms, postnasal drip, acid reflux, and partially-chewed food.

Sometimes you cough because you're breathing in dry air. I hear about this in my clinic from runners and others who exercise outdoors: this transient type of cough disappears without causing harm. Breathing in dry air longterm can be both annoyingly troublesome and potentially harmful to the **airway mucosa** (the moist mucous membranes protecting the airway from outside irritants).

At other times we're coughing up **mucus,** consisting of water, salt and various proteins that help trap germs and particles of dirt. A layer of microscopic hairy, towel-like cells called **cilia** moves the mucus up and out toward the back of the throat.

Coughing is a reflex (a neurological response) similar to the pain reflex that's "hard-wired" into the marvelous complexity of our brains. All reflexes are "wired" to receptors in different parts of the body. These receptors work like tiny pickup microphones designed to respond to specific stimuli such as dust, acid, pressure, sound and other irritants. Once a stimulus is picked up by the receptors, that information is transmitted to the processing center in the brain through "wires" that run through the spine. Yes, our system is wired, my friends. We do not have Bluetooth wireless reflexes!

One set of these wires, otherwise known as nerves, brings the message of the stimulus to the brain's **cough center,** which then sends an outgoing message through another set of "nerve-wires." This message goes to the lungs, diaphragm, muscles, and ribs, telling them to "cough, cough, cough."

The cough center is very connected to the brain's emotional center, because the nerve between the cough center and the diaphragm passes through it. This is why strong emotions can cause a cough, as explained in Chapter 5; emotional stress can even trigger an asthma attack, and stress can also increase acid reflux, another trigger for coughs.

The **diaphragm**, a thin layer of muscle dividing the belly from the chest, responds by pulling down the chest and the lungs—like two flexible "sponges" inside the chest—which then fill up with air. This is called the in-breath or inspiratory phase of a cough. In a matter of milliseconds the cannon of your lungs is ready to fire. The diaphragm is very

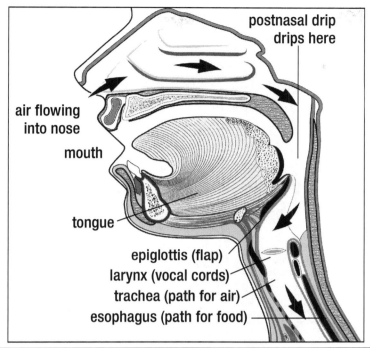

air flowing
into nose

postnasal drip
drips here

mouth

tongue

epiglottis (flap)
larynx (vocal cords)
trachea (path for air)
esophagus (path for food)

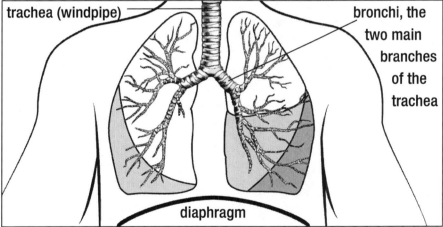

trachea (windpipe)

bronchi, the
two main
branches
of the
trachea

diaphragm

impatient and does not wait for the flap in the throat (the epiglottis) to open. It fires with the epiglottis-flap closed at the top of the throat, generating even higher and more explosive pressures. The flap can't contain the pressure from the cannon of the lungs, and it blows open (the "expulsive phase" of the cough). Typically, most if not all the offending particles or elements will fly out, riding on thousands of saliva droplets at speeds up to 20 miles an hour.

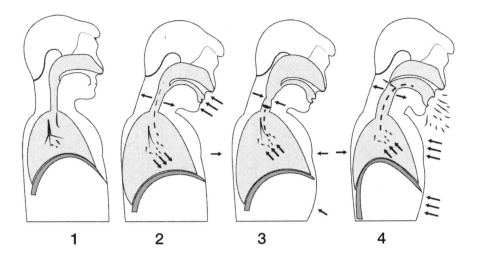

The four stages of a cough:
  1. irritation
  2. inspiration
  3. compression
  4. expulsion.

In the compression phase, note the flap of the epiglottis closing, then the epiglottis blowing open from the force of the cough in the expulsion phase.

It's impressive that the body can clear the lungs with such great speed and pressure, but the results of repeated coughing—especially violent coughing—can also include exhaustion, insomnia, headache, dizziness, rib pain, hoarseness, sweating, and urinary incontinence. A severe cough can generate up to 500 pounds of pressure which can fracture ribs, a rare but painful and potentially serious complication. The ribs most likely to fracture are the middle ones, on the outside of the chest, and people with osteoporosis are most vulnerable.

Coughing is a symptom, not a disease. Coughing is our body's response to an attack by some source, whether pollen, an environmental irritant like smoke, or mucus brought on by an infection. The attack could be mild or serious. Whether a cough is caused by an infection or an environmental irritant, it's typically accompanied by a stuffy, runny nose—in other words, it can be hard to tell whether you have a cold or an allergy. (When you have a cold, you have malaise and possibly muscle pain. In other words you feel sick all over and you are more likely to have a profuse, non-stop runny nose.)

A cold is one of the most common causes of a cough, so the two often go together. To me, as a doctor, a common cold is not a disease at all. It is a transient state of imbalance, something disturbing the body's **homeostasis** (its tendency to return to normal when out of whack). This imbalance is a passing state. Having a cold is normal: every human being on the whole planet will experience a common cold, at some moment in life, if not annually. Even in the tropical heat of Cuba, people catch colds!

When a cough is caused by an infection, it's usually viral, because **viruses** cause colds and most flu-like illnesses. (**Bacteria** can also cause coughs associated with sinusitis, strep throat and other infections.) There are hundreds of different kinds of viruses, and each virus species has multiple variations. Imagine that a virus is like a chameleon: when exposed to green leaves chameleons become green but if they move to a brown branch they will become brownish. Viruses are very similar, constantly changing their coats. Not only are there hundreds of possible viruses, but viruses mutate from year to year, creating ever-new strains we need to be protected from. It takes years to develop a new drug, which means it is difficult for drugs to keep up with the new viruses.

Double pneumonia, walking pneumonia—what's the difference?

Now that we've learned about the causes of coughs, let's learn about some specific disease states associated with coughs.

Pneumonia is an infection in the lungs. It occurs when a virus, bacterium or fungus breaks through our defenses in the lining of the breathing system (from the tip of the nose all the way down into the lungs). Our body never gives up, however, and it attempts to control the invaders with an inflammatory reaction. When the reaction occurs in the lungs, the **alveoli** (all the little sacs that form the lungs) fill up with a fluid to protect them. This fluid contains microscopic fragments of the lungs and organisms lost in our internal battlefield. We tend to cough it out as green, yellowish, or even dark brown **sputum**. (**Phlegm** is thick mucus in the nose, throat or lungs; once it's spit out, it's called **sputum** or **expectoration.**)

Pneumonia patients have symptoms such as a persistent fever (more than three days), a productive cough (with phlegm), shortness of breath and sometimes **wheezes** (doctors' term for wheezy noises coming from the lung). The doctor can hear **crackles,** a crackly sound with the stethoscope, similar to the sound of rubbing your hair between your fingers close to your ears. The chest X-ray usually shows a diffuse whitish shadow (see illustrations below).

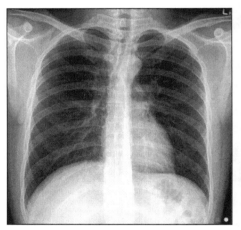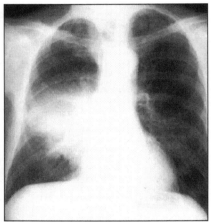

A clear chest X-ray (left) and an X-ray of lungs with pneumonia (right). See whitish shadow on the left side of the second X-ray.

Children under five, the elderly and people with a weak immune system are most likely to get a severe case of pneumonia and possibly even die from it. Nearly a million children died from pneumonia worldwide in 2015, while in the US a total of about 50,000 people of all ages died.

Walking pneumonia: People with a mild case of pneumonia may have so few symptoms that they can go to work and otherwise "walk around" with it. The symptoms are the same as a cold or flu, and in fact doctors will not diagnose it as pneumonia until they order a chest X-ray and see the whitish shadow caused by the fluid in the lungs (see X-ray samples). What most people call "walking pneumonia," a physician will diagnose as "atypical pneumonia."

So how would you even know to go to your doctor about possible pneumonia? The biggest clue is that the symptoms keep getting worse after three or four days. If they start getting better, you have a cold or flu. Longer than that, you might have pneumonia. Definitely see your doctor if you have one or more of the symptoms listed on page 23.

Double pneumonia: Intuition to the contrary, this does not mean that you have two types of bacteria or two types of viruses. It means you have pneumonia in both lungs, usually caused by the same organism.

Pneumonia, bronchitis or asthma? It's up to your doctor to diagnose these conditions; here we'll just explain the difference. Pneumonia is an infection in the lungs, while bronchitis has similar symptoms but the infection is in the **bronchi** (the branching tubes leading from the trachea or windpipe to the lungs). Asthma is a genetic predisposition triggered by an infection or allergens, and it involves inflammation plus narrowing of the airways that cause the typical wheezing when the person breathes out. While pneumonia and bronchitis last longer than a cold or acute cough — typically weeks longer — asthma can last for years. People with asthma can get pneumonia; they are not exempt!

Sinusitis is an infection in the sinuses, the empty air-filled spaces in our face alongside and above our nose. Like pneumonia, it is an inflammatory response to a breakthrough of the defense mechanism by a bacteria or virus. Some common sinusitis symptoms are typical of the flu and of other upper respiratory infections, including a productive (mucus-producing) cough, headache, and possibly a low-grade fever.

The person may have pain in one or both ears, which could also indicate an ear infection. But one symptom clearly tells us that the person has sinusitis: pain when a finger is pressed on the bones above or below the eyes or alongside the nose. It's possible to have sinusitis without this symptom, but if you have it, you definitely have sinusitis. You can test this for yourself: see the illustrations on the next page.

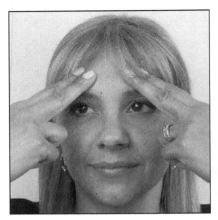
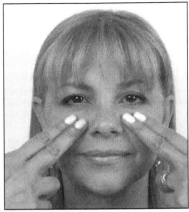

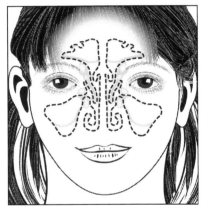

Palpating the sinuses above and below the eyes to check for sinusitis; (below) sinuses are hollow areas above, below and beside the nose.

Sepsis occurs when bacteria or viruses invade the blood. The invaders enter through a hole in the "city walls" (the skin or the mucosal lining of the airways). If our disease fighters—the battalion of macrophages (scavenger cells)—cannot contain the invading forces, they will use our own cells to multiply themselves. At some point they reach the blood circulation "highways" and will go to every corner of our body.

In the blood highways they will encounter our body's Marine Corps and other key defense battalions. The bacteria overcome by our defenses will release toxic fragments, causing the added symptoms of low blood pressure, headache, confusion, and dehydration. If the body does not get antibiotics to help contain this bacterial septic state, death is quite possible. Viruses can produce a severe pneumonia and blood sepsis, but unfortunately they will not respond to antibiotics, and antiviral drugs are of limited help.

Mild viral infections can be treated at home with the natural remedies described in Chapters 4 to 7. Sometimes serious viral infections like the H1N1 flu of several years ago cause respiratory distress so severe that people can die from it. These patients end up in an Intensive Care Unit like the one where I work, where we provide supportive treatment: mechanical ventilation assists with breathing, and if the blood pressure is low we provide oral or intravenous fluids to bring it back up again. Basically, we support the body through the process of attack, hoping that the patient's own defenses will finally contain and destroy the invaders. Patients usually survive, but only if the problems are diagnosed quickly and treated effectively, rapidly and knowledgeably.

Common colds, the major cause of acute coughs, are caused by viruses and very seldom caused by bacteria. When viruses attack our body, they go into our cells where antibiotics generally can't reach them. Antibiotics are specifically designed to kill or neutralize bacteria (which live *outside* our cells), so these drugs really should be called "antibacterials." Antivirals are designed to attack viruses, but they are only partially effective and even then only when given within the first few hours.

An acute cough rarely lasts more than three weeks, with symptoms typically beginning with mucus and ending with a dry cough. It's absolutely normal for a persistent nagging cough to last for three weeks. Acute cough characteristics (wet or dry, with or without post nasal drip) change as the virus interacts with the body's defenses. Our amazing organism will respond to the viral attack by generating symptoms as reactions to the damage produced by the battle. For this very reason the "all-in-one" treatment idea in most over-the-counter medications simply does not work. The treatment should be specific, targeting the specific phase of the battle. We don't want to use to fight a war when a diplomatic conversation can resolve the problem.

Although it's not a cause for alarm, an acute cough can be trouble-some and bothersome. So in the next few chapters we will explore natural ways to alleviate the symptoms, shorten the duration, and improve your quality of life.

❧ FOUR ❧

Grandma's Favorites:
Steams and Gargles, Soups and Teas

As the wind blows from the southern part of the bay, it caresses the leaves of the octogenarian mango trees on my grandpa's farm in Palmar, Cuba. This sweet little old man used to get up at six o'clock every morning to feed his chickens and tend to his trees, rain or shine. Grandma Juana was never too far behind. She too would wake at the crack of dawn and make her way to the kitchen to start her morning ritual—cafésito Cubano.

I remember one cloudy morning while visiting them for the weekend; grandma and I were making a delicious café-con-leche *in the kitchen when from the back porch we heard a thunderous cough, followed by frequent efforts to clear the throat. It was grandpa; it seemed that three days of 70° "winter" weather was enough to affect his health. Next thing we heard was, "Juana, can you please make me a tamarind tea? I think I'm catching a cold," followed by more throat-clearing attempts.*

Grandma replied in her sweet voice, "Sure, but you have to give me a minute, I have to go get the leaves from the tree." She went out back and returned as fast as her little 80-year-old legs could carry her. "Would you like honey in your tea?" she lovingly asked him.

"Absolutely. Honey is the elixir of life. When you get to be 100 years old in this town, honey practically runs through your veins!"

Grandpa had a great sense of humor — we all had a chuckle. Grandma put the leaves to boil in the oldest pot I'd ever seen. Passed down from her mom, it was over 75 years old. After 15 minutes, the soothing aroma permeated the tiny two bedroom house. Once the tea was ready, she shuffled to the bedroom where grandpa had gone to lie down. In one hand she had her jarrito *(cup) filled with tamarind tea while the other hand held three fresh sage leaves for him to chew on to soothe his throat.*

This combination of natural remedies and teas was the pharmacy I grew up with. Back home no one ever went to the doctor for acute coughs or colds. By the age of ten I was pretty familiar with all the most common remedies around. As it turned out, good ol' grandma lived to be 94 and grandpa 102 years old, God bless their souls, and they hardly ever went to a doctor.

Fifty years ago, the medical industry experienced a substantial shift. The great pharmaceutical companies surfaced. The treatment of diseases moved from the empirical use of tinctures and teas to pills and injections. Undoubtedly, modern pharmaceuticals have brought about great improvements in the practice of medicine with a significant prolongation of life. But teas and home remedies fell out of favor, considered ineffective and possibly unsafe. Thus the wealth of knowledge about herbal medicine, acquired over thousands of years, was lost within two generations. Using pharmaceutical drugs became a sign of scientific progress, and herbal remedies became a thing of the past. Many of my patients, especially the Hispanics and African Americans, are nostalgic about their grandmothers preparing healing teas from the backyard herb garden. They regret that no one learned from grandma while she was still alive.

Today, I have no doubt that pharmaceutical products bring value to the practice of medicine. However, physicians should not neglect the significance of herbal remedies for the treatment of acute cough. In fact, herbal remedies are the foundation of the pharmaceutical industry. Many of our most powerful drugs were made from traditional herbs, such as aspirin from white willow bark, digitalis from foxglove, colchicine from autumn crocus, atropine from belladonna, and even muscle relaxants from the Amazon rainforest herbs in curare. I would never use herbal teas or tinctures in the Intensive Care Unit, but for a common cold or flu, natural remedies should be the cornerstone of your home medicine cabinet. In this chapter I'll describe the most valuable remedies made from ingredients commonly available in most kitchens, while the next chapter will involve a trip to your local health food store.

Differences between herbal medicines and OTC drugs

Since the beginning of time, humans have used plants as medicine. In the last 150 years, since the Bayer Company first isolated and synthesized aspirin from white willow bark, the pharmaceutical industry has focused on isolating the active ingredient in medicinal plants (the chemical producing the desired effect) so that it could be made more powerful and the dosage level could be controlled for safety. Once the active ingredient was isolated, it could also be made synthetically in the lab, thereby ensuring quality control.

One problem with this approach is that the higher the concentration, the greater the likelihood of side effects. Another is the failure to use other possible medicinal substances in the plants. As Dr. Andrew Weil has explained, "We forget about the plant. We don't study any of the other compounds in it or their complex interactions." With these other active ingredients left out, the synthetic version is not only less effective than the original plant, it lacks substances which could modulate any toxic effects of the main active ingredient. The result is drugs that have far worse side effects than could be expected from simply making the active ingredient stronger.

These harmful side effects might be tolerable if the synthetic drug's benefits were proportionately greater. But as Dr. Weil has stated, "Single-agent (isolated active ingredient) drugs would be acceptable if they actually yielded better results. But the fact is that the natural whole plant often has both benefits and safety that puts the isolated compounds to shame."

This particular statement especially holds true for treating acute cough.

My fellow pulmonologists in Europe recognize the value of home remedies in acute coughs and colds. In 2001 the World Health Organization, composed primarily of European physicians, issued a white paper entitled *Cough and Cold Remedies for the Treatment of Acute Respiratory Infection in Young Children* which concluded, "There is no reason to believe that a safe, soothing home-made remedy is less effective than a safe commercial remedy. Home remedies are usually inexpensive and promote self-reliance. Unlike commercial preparations, which may contain potentially harmful ingredients, most homemade remedies are harmless."

The foundational principles of our *Cough Cures* are effectiveness, accuracy, safety and simplicity. It is supported by research on the effectiveness of natural remedies. I know it can be overwhelming to select the appropriate treatment, with so many over-the-counter and natural remedies to choose from. We've tried to simplify the choice by suggesting the most effective natural remedies, whether you prefer making your own in the kitchen or searching online or in the health food store (next chapter). You can delve into each chapter for the details or skip right to the shortcut guide at the end.

Nothing Like Grandma's Healing Touch

Let's explore some of grandma's favorite homemade remedies.

Lemon and honey "cough syrup"

This is one of the most popular traditional homemade remedies, used throughout different cultures for centuries. Honey and lemon are common foods that are surprisingly medicinal. They're especially soothing for coughs. Here's a simple way to make a hot honey-lemonade that you can keep sipping all day to keep hydrated and thin your mucus, making it easier to clear out of your system. Or you can use this drink as a honey-lemon gargle.

Put a cup of water (125 ml) on to boil. Meantime, squeeze half a lemon, but first, roll it hard back and forth with the flat of your hand to break it down and make it easier to juice. When the water is hot (not quite boiling), pour it through the lemon juicer to get as much of the pulp and juice as possible.

Add a spoonful of honey to taste, if you like. Manuka honey is best if you're sick (it has the strongest antimicrobial properties) although it's also the most expensive. Or use local honey if you can find it. Best to avoid supermarket honey, which is often cut with sugar or high fructose corn syrup.

Variations

Lemon seeds: Throughout the Caribbean, the lemon seeds are boiled in the lemon water. Although we don't have research to document the medicinal effect, such a widespread practice is likely to be have some basis in fact, since they are clearly not added for flavor — they make the lemon water quite bitter.

Lime drink: The juice of a lime can be substituted for half a lemon, and either one can be drunk without honey. Using hot water takes the edge off the sourness and makes a very pleasant drink even without sweetening.

Honey water: Honey has antioxidant, antiviral and antibacterial properties. Honey may help eliminate the secondary bacterial infections that can come with colds and flu. Interestingly, honey scored better than dextromethorphan (an active ingredient in Robitussin) in a research study* comparing how well they worked for children's night time coughs!

You can stir honey to taste into tea or hot water. One caveat, don't give honey to infants and children under two years of age as it may be contaminated with botulism spores and they can develop botulism.

Ginger drink

Ginger roots are widely used for the treatment of coughs. Studies have documented its wide variety of medicinal uses, including its effectiveness against RSV, a respiratory virus that affects babies. Moms all over the world, from India to Jamaica, use ginger for acute coughs. Ginger can be either chewed or boiled. However, boiled and ingested as a tea is the method most commonly used and studied.

The Dr. Gus method: Boil two one-inch (.5 cm) pieces of peeled ginger root in 32 oz. (1 liter) of water for 15 minutes. You can add a little lemon juice plus honey or raw blue agave nectar to sweeten.

Burke prefers simmering thinly-sliced ginger and makes Indian chai by adding black tea, cinnamon and cardamom (each with its own medicinal properties). Strain and add milk to taste, or as she prefers, a plant-based milk substitute such as almond milk.

Tamarind drink

This is not only one of my favorites from childhood, it is actually recommended by the World Health Organization in its *Cough and Cold Remedies for the Treatment of Acute Respiratory Infection in Young Children.*

Boil two tablespoons (30 to 40 gm) of finely chopped tamarind leaves in 16 oz. (250 ml) of water for 15 minutes. Then strain. Consider adding a little lemon juice and honey or raw blue agave nectar to sweeten. WHO recommends two cups a day, however in my hometown people drink it freely, as much as they want.

---

*See Appendix D for research on the ingredients in this chapter, and the Endnotes for research not specifically related to one substance.

Green tea, black tea and **coffee** contain bacteria-killing substances. You wouldn't give them to a child but you can certainly enjoy their medicinal properties yourself.

If you want to make your own cough syrup, try a blend of honey and a surprising herb: **coffee.** (Yes, coffee is an herbal medicine because caffeine has a powerful effect on the human body, including dilating the air passageways in the lungs.) Recent research demonstrated that a jam-like paste of honey and instant coffee was highly effective against lingering coughs, while the standard medication, prednisolone, had little effect!

Fresh garlic (organic if possible): Chop a good size clove fairly fine and add a tablespoon of honey. Swallow without chewing; repeat every 2-4 hours. If you notice that this method gives you an upset stomach, try garlic capsules instead. Odorless garlic caps are available at health food stores or online.

H$_2$O and you — oral hydration and mist therapy

Postnasal drip (excess mucus production dripping down behind the nose and throat during acute viral infection) is one of the most common triggers of acute coughs. We need the layer of mucus for protection, to move germs and foreign particles out of the nose and throat, but too much of it is a mechanical irritant triggering a cough. Drinking plenty of water and exposing your face to water vapors can liquefy mucus, including postnasal drip, and help you cough it out or blow it out your nose.

There are several ways to deliver water vapors, including sophisticated systems with nozzles. However, you accomplish the same results by boiling a quart (liter) of water and adding a teaspoon (10 gm) of salt. Once boiling, remove from heat and put your face close enough to inhale the vapors.

Do not cover a child's head with a towel or get too close to try to maximize the effect. This may burn the tissue that lines the nostrils, throat and lower respiratory system producing inflammation and worsening the mucus production.

Oral hydration

This is fancy doctor-talk for drinking a lot of water! I find that when I examine the inside of my patients' noses and throats, I often find dried mucus, especially in the winter when the air is dry from the heating system. Simply drinking more water is helpful for restoring healthy moisture to the protective mucous membranes. It's *remotely* possible that too much water can lower your sodium in a dangerous way, so it's safer not to drink more than 10 glasses (2.5 liters) of fluids per day. (Of course you need more if you are sweating a lot from heat or exercise.) Your fluids should be mostly water, not coffee, which tends to act as a diuretic (in other words, coffee stimulates your body to get rid of water by urinating).

Saline nasal rinses are effective in softening dry or thick nasal mucus. They can improve cold symptoms — primarily sneezing, stuffy nose and sore throat — but they do not shorten the duration of a cold. My favorite is Xlear (pronounced "clear"), a saline rinse enhanced with xylitol—a well-researched natural substance that helps kill germs, reduce swelling inside the nose, and prevent biofilm. My patients report great results with Xlear, whereas they often complain of burning with conventional saline.

Don't use any nasal rinse for more than two weeks, even though some rinses recommend daily use as a preventive measure. The mucus inside your nose creates a protective barrier, so extended daily use can actually increase your risk of infection by depleting this barrier.

A bulb syringe is better for kids because it will add gentle pressure. The Mayo Clinic's website (www.mayoclinic.com) has helpful instructional videos for using a bulb syringe. You can safely use saline nasal drops for children with nasal congestion, particularly when it interferes with breastfeeding. They come packaged with a little bulb syringe for babies, which you can use to suction the mucus from the baby's nose.

No pharmacy near by? No worries, you can make your own saline solution. Put a cup of water to boil. Add a quarter teaspoon of salt, stir until salt is dissolved, and let it cool. Pour into a clean plastic nasal spray bottle, available inexpensively at any pharmacy. I hope you kept yours from the last time you needed one!

You can also use a NeilMed plastic squeeze bottle prefilled with saline solution. I only recommend this brand because it takes care of two serious problems with generic saline squeeze bottles: it has a bulb at the tip to control the flow, to protect against the water flowing in under too much pressure; and the slightly acidic saline solution has been buffered to prevent the acidity from irritating the nasal passages.

For more complete clearing of the nasal passages, use a **neti pot,** a little ceramic or plastic pot with a spout that directs warm salt water into one of your nostrils, to be flushed out the other. The saline solution clears out cough-inducing allergens and mucus, including postnasal drip. Neti pots are available in drug stores and health food stores, and you can find demonstrations of how to use them on YouTube. Both Xlear and NeilMed make neti pots that come with their special solutions. Be sure to use distilled water, not tap water, which has on rare occasions introduced an infection via the nostrils.

Lean forward and tilt your head slightly to one side and allow the saline solution to gently flow in through one nostril and out the other. Make sure your tongue sits on the roof of your mouth to prevent it from coming out through your mouth.

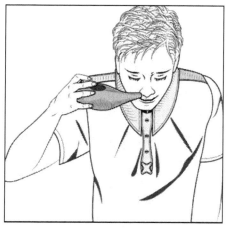
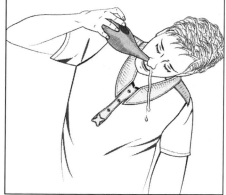

Gargles

Saline: Research has proven that a simple water or saline (salted water) gargle every one to two hours during initial cold/flu symptoms such as a sore throat is a highly effective preventive measure. For example, make a salt water gargle with half a teaspoon of salt in a full glass of warm water (gargle for a few seconds then spit it out). Researchers in Japan found that people who gargled with warm water three times a day during the cold and flu season (a popular health habit in Japan) had a nearly 40 percent decrease in upper respiratory tract infections. If they did get sick, they had fewer bronchial symptoms. Salt water is likely to be even more effective than the plain warm water used in the Japanese research.

A saline gargle is especially effective when flying, because people tend to get sick easily on planes from the dry air drying out the protective mucus in their nose/throat area. Research has shown that gargling once an hour is a great way to prevent the colds and coughs that people often catch while flying.

Romerillo is a medicinal plant with little white flowers, popular with Hispanics. You can easily find it in any backyard in the Southeast. The leaves are made into an herbal tea to treat coughs, sore throats, stuffy and runny noses by Hispanics for centuries. If you live in the south and haven't used romerillo yet, ask a Hispanic neighbor to show you where it grows!

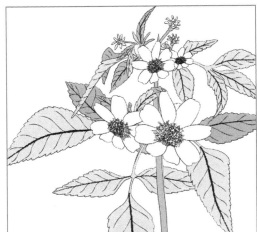

Preparation: Boil a quart (liter) of water. Remove from heat, add five to seven stems of romerillo with the leaves (no roots or flowers), and cover. Cool until it reaches room temperature, then strain. Add a teaspoon of honey and few drops of lemon.

Gargle every four hours. You may also drink this as a tea, but only consume every eight hours.

Chest rubs: You can rub Vicks VapoRub on your child's chest where she can safely inhale the vapors. You can also rub it on her feet or put a swipe above the upper lip. Just make sure the goop doesn't get up her nose where it can be inhaled. A research study in *Pediatrics* documented that this type of rub helps reduce congestion and nighttime coughing. Get some sleep!

Superfoods from grandma's kitchen (you're in for a treat!)

When you are sick, focus on eating superfoods. You may not have much of an appetite, which means that everything you eat or drink has to count for a lot! It has to be really nutrient dense; in other words, you want to get the maximum possible nutrients from the smallest amount of food. Here are some ways to do that:

Incorporate fruits, especially berries, mangos and citrus because they are high in vitamin C and bioflavonoids. Once you have recovered your appetite, I recommend a diet based on steamed vegetables with baked or steamed fish and poultry. Stay away from fatty and junk foods, because they promote inflammation and lack the nutrients needed to fight infection.

Raw vegetable juices extract the nutrients and make them really easy to digest, at a time when your body does not have a lot of energy for digesting.

Garlic is like nature's antibiotic and antiviral. Taste too strong for you? Mince it and add it to the honey-lemon tea above (it's surprisingly palatable that way) or add to salsa, tomato sauce, guacamole, or hummus.

Chocolate is one of my favorite traditional medicines! Recent research shows it reduces heart attacks and strokes; however it works for other things too. Theobromine, a chemical component of chocolate, is a natural cough suppressant. The darker the chocolate, the higher the concentration of theobromine: unsweetened dark chocolate has 450 mg of theobromine per ounce, while sweetened dark chocolate has only a third of that amount and milk chocolate has only a sixth as much.

You can have one to two ounces of dark chocolate a day (make sure you buy it with at least 70% cocoa and minimal sweetening). As tempting as it may be, don't overdo it. Excessive consumption of chocolate may interfere with your sleep, as chocolate also contains caffeine.

Plant-based dairy products: Switch to almond milk, rice milk, or other plant-based milk products, because cow's milk may worsen your postnasal drip and cough. Research studies show that soymilk has the same effect as cow's milk. Almond milk can be a wonderful substitute. My family uses almond milk because we have found that one of my daughters gets congested from cow's milk, even though she is not lactose intolerant.

Grandma Lina's preferred diet — soup

Liquids are best during the first few days of a cold, especially when you have no appetite. Liquids help hydrate and thin your mucus, thus making it easier to cough it out. Drink liquids such as water, orange juice, lemonade, herbal teas and hot broths. Avoid sugary drinks and juices. (Fresh orange juice is best, not bottled or from concentrate, and definitely without added sugars).

Homemade chicken soup really does have immune-enhancing properties — grandma was right! In fact its effectiveness was documented in a study published in the journal of the American College of Chest Physicians. And it was published in the issue containing the best articles in the organization's 75-year history! (This was a major exception to my observation that physicians' professional associations and journals fail to focus on common, everyday ailments.)

The study showed the effect of chicken soup on neutrophils, the immune system cells in the bloodstream which the body mobilizes to defend itself against viral infections like colds and flu. Neutrophils stimulate the formation of large amounts of mucus, the most common cause of acute coughs. This study proved in vitro (in the laboratory) that chicken soup inhibits the neutrophils, thus reducing excess mucus and indirectly alleviating coughs. It also proved that homemade soup is superior to any canned soup on the market. Way to go, grandma!

Every family has its own traditional way of preparing chicken soup, which we pretty much all refer to as "grandma's chicken soup." This is the recipe from my mother — my children's "Grandma Lina" — very similar to the recipe published in the journal.

Ingredients

1 5 to 6 lb. (2 to 3 kg) stewing hen or baking chicken

1 package of chicken wings

3 large onions

1 large sweet potato

3 parsnips

11 or 12 large carrots

5 or 6 celery stems

1 bunch of parsley

salt and pepper to taste

Preparation

Clean the chicken, put it in a large pot, and cover it with cold water. Bring the water to a boil. Add the chicken wings and chopped root vegetables. Boil about 1.5 hours. Remove fat from the surface as it accumulates. Add the parsley and celery. Cook the mixture about 45 minutes longer. Remove the chicken. The chicken is not used further for the soup. (The meat makes excellent chicken parmesan.) Puree the vegetables in a food processor, then add them back to the broth if you want a thick soup. People who are quite ill may prefer the simple broth without the vegetables. Salt and pepper to taste. Note: this soup freezes well.

The recipe in the journal came from a Jewish grandma, therefore matzoh balls were added to the soup. But in my house, chicken soup was not complete unless it contained *malanga,* also known as taro or *yautia* (an edible tropical root).

Fire Cider: How about making a potent cough-and-cold-deflecting, nasal-passage clearing, chest-congestion-releasing brew out of ingredients you have in your kitchen (or can easily get)? Fire Cider is a traditional recipe with many variations. It tastes much better than it sounds! The idea of horseradish turns a lot of people off, but that's what really opens up your sinuses. You can buy Fire Cider bottled at your health food store, however Rosemary Gladstar (the godmother of modern herbal medicine in America and the one who concocted this recipe) encourages everyone to make their own as a form of "people's medicine."

Here's her recipe, with a few added comments from us.

1 part fresh horseradish root

1 part onions

1 part garlic

1/2 part fresh ginger

Cayenne to taste (just a few grains will do).*

Honey to taste

Apple cider vinegar

Optional ingredients: turmeric, echinacea, cinnamon, etc.

* To taste means the brew should be hot, but not so hot you can't tolerate it. Better to make it a little milder than too hot; you can always add more cayenne pepper later if necessary.

Chop fresh garlic, onions, and horseradish into small pieces and grate fresh ginger. You can put all the ingredients in a food processor to protect yourself against the eye-stinging experience of chopping them.

The amounts don't have to be precise and will vary according to your particular taste. If unsure, start with equal amounts of the first three ingredients and roughly half part ginger the first time you make this; you can always adjust the flavors in future batches. Chop enough of the first four ingredients to fill a quart jar approximately half full. Put in wide mouth quart jar and cover with apple cider vinegar to about two to three inches above the herbs. You want raw unpasteurized vinegar with "mother of vinegar" lurking murkily in the bottom, readily available in health food stores.

Add cayenne to taste, just a small amount or it will be too hot!. Let sit in a warm place for two to four weeks (the longer is sits, the stronger the results). Best to shake every day to help extract the medicinal properties from the herbs. Before using, strain and discard spent herbs.

Add honey to taste. Warm the honey first so it mixes in well. "A spoonful of honey helps the medicine go down…" Honey not only tempers the spicy flavor, it adds its own medicinal properties.

Your Fire Cider should taste hot, spicy, and sweet. Rebottle and enjoy! Fire Cider will keep for several months unrefrigerated if stored in a cool pantry, but it's better to store in the refrigerator if you have room. A small shot glass daily serves as an excellent tonic, or take frequent teaspoons if you feel a cold coming on. Take it as frequently as necessary to strengthen your immune system.

Your Shortcut Guide to Grandma's Favorites

You're bound to have at least a few of these in your kitchen:
- fresh-squeezed lemon juice in hot water
- honey
- garlic or ginger
- apple cider vinegar (dilute a little in water)
- salt water for a saline gargle or nasal flush
- dark chocolate
- chicken soup, preferably home made
- Vicks Vaporub for a chest or foot rub

If you live in the south, you might find fresh tamarind or romerillo leaves in your back yard like my Grandma Juana did!

Don't forget to drink plenty of water and use a nasal rinse when needed (a neti pot or saline spray) — my favorites are NeilMed and Xlear.

The Proof Is in the Pudding:
Evidence-Based Herbs and Supplements

Long before the dawn of recorded history, a man, two women, and a baby were buried in the cave that was their home, their grave decorated with pine boughs interlaced with the wildflowers of the surrounding hills. These flowers — varieties of hollyhock and ephedra, yarrow and groundsel — are used to this day by the local villagers as medicine.

The time? 50,000 years ago, give or take 10,000 years.

The place? A Neanderthal cave in Kurdistan unearthed by Columbia University archeologists.

The evidence? Pollen analysis of the soil around the graves, showing clusters of pollen that could not have been just blown in by the wind.

The first known medicines were herbs used by Neanderthals some 50,000 years ago.

Herbs are as old as the hills and as current as modern chemistry techniques. Their vitamins and minerals, their antioxidants and phytonutrients have been extracted and isolated, offering modern sufferers the option of using concentrated supplements instead of herbs. In the last chapter we talked about natural cough remedies so simple you can find the ingredients in your kitchen. Now let's foray farther afield, to your local health food store, for other natural options for treating coughs — herbs, supplements, and medicinal foods.

We often hear that these natural products are "unproven." In many cases there is research to support a product, but it was done overseas and was not included in your physician's training. In other cases, the evidence comes from practitioners' experience with the products, or—in the case of herbs—from hundreds or even thousands of years of traditional usage. Appendix D lists research studies for the herbs and supplements we recommend.

Food is often the best medicine, and one of the best ways to cram a lot of good nutrition into one meal is a breakfast smoothie with a very good greens powder like Green Vibrance from Vibrant Health, which has a long and astonishing list of organic ingredients. For a fabulous breakfast, put a scoopful in the blender with protein powder (un-denatured whey protein or Garden of Life vegan), maybe half a cup of berries (frozen, if you like your smoothie chilled), and some fish oil, plus enough water for your desired consistency. To add some warmth in the winter, you could use almond butter, cacao, ginger and cinnamon.

Let's say you don't always eat a perfect diet. You'll need supplements for overall health, as well as to treat and prevent coughs, especially during cold and flu season. Get yourself a good-quality multivitamin supplement (preferably a natural brand rather than a drugstore brand because they use inferior-quality synthetic vitamins). Don't waste your money on a one-a-day; it just isn't possible to fit everything you need into one pill. These vitamins do so many things in your body, they're a good investment.

A good multi will contain enough of most nutrients to supplement a reasonably healthy diet, although you'll need other vitamins separately because multis don't contain enough of them. Let's look at just a few. I find if I try to take too many pills, I get overwhelmed, give up and don't take anything. I don't want that to happen to you! Here are my priorities.

Vitamin D: Most people need to supplement this vitamin, especially in the winter when you're not going outside and getting it from sunlight. If you're not sure you need it, ask your physician for a blood test (it must be the 25[OH]D test) or get a home test from the Vitamin D Research Council, www.vitamindcouncil.org. See Dr. Mark Hyman's blog on vitamin D at www.drhyman.com for the amount to supplement. Be sure to get vitamin D_3 (not D_2 which most doctors prescribe). It will help your health in many ways in addition to preventing coughs, colds, even asthma.

Essential fatty acids from fish oil were shown in recent research to be as effective as Singulair in treating exercise-induced asthma episodes. Essential fatty acids, especially omega-3 fats, are extremely important for your immune system as well as for hormone balancing, preventing inflammation, and many other health benefits. Yet they are difficult to get from the average American diet, which has harmful fats (like fried foods and trans fats) that actually work *against* the healthy ones.

You can get healthy fats from avocado, walnuts, and fish. Avoid farmed fish, which lack these nutrients, as well as mercury-tainted fish like swordfish. Or supplement with fish oil, krill oil, or plant-based essential fatty acids. Nordic Naturals and Carlson are excellent brands for fish oils. My fave? Barlean's Chocolate Raspberry Swirl!

Probiotics are the friendly bacteria that live in your digestive system. Like essential fatty acids, they can be harmed by the typical American lifestyle (in this case, by antibiotics and other drugs, sugar and artificial sweeteners, and the chlorine and fluoride in tap water). You can help your friendly gut bacteria with fermented foods (yogurt with live cultures, kefir, kombucha, and *refrigerated* pickles and sauerkraut) or with probiotic supplements. Fermented foods are easy to make at home and can also be found in larger health food stores. Look for probiotics with a wide range of organisms and a high bacteria count (billions, not millions, of organisms). My favorite brands: Jarrow, Garden of Life, Renew Life.

To help your gut bacteria flourish, you'll also need good fiber, specifically *soluble* fiber from fruits and oats, beans and peas, and one of my all-time favorite medicinal foods, **chia seeds.** Soak a teaspoon of these tiny black seeds in a cup of water overnight and watch them jelly up. Add to a smoothie or cereal for help with your digestion, immune system, diabetes, cardiovascular health and many other health conditions.

Magnesium is the most important mineral that most Americans are deficient in. So important for coughs! In fact magnesium administered intravenously in the ER for kids with asthma attacks provided "remarkable improvement" in one research study and allowed these kids to be discharged home instead of being admitted to the hospital. Why wait for an asthma attack? Make sure you and your kids are getting enough magnesium. My favorite way: Natural Calm, a fruit-flavored drink powder. It also helps with anxiety and insomnia, because magnesium helps your brain relax along with any tense, cramping or spasmodic muscles.

Zinc keeps your immune system strong. Zinc lozenges (made with the specific form of zinc that will send zinc ions up into your nose) prevent cold viruses from replicating and shorten the duration of a cold, cough or sinus infection. The best brands include Cold-Eeze and Zand. The latter has a myriad of flavors of cough drops providing zinc plus herbs, with natural sweeteners. (For a few days when you're sick it's safe to take 150 to 200 mg a day of zinc, but not long-term as it can create a copper deficiency.)

A good all-around **immune formula** like Source Naturals' Wellness Formula will contain many of the vitamins and minerals just mentioned, plus more than a dozen of the herbs for coughs we're about to meet in the next section. Source Naturals is an excellent supplement brand in general, along with Natural Factors and Jarrow.

Three more special supplements have antimicrobial properties for when you do get sick.

Oil of oregano worked well against severe bacterial infections, including antibiotic-resistant bacteria like the hospital super-bug MRSA, in a research study which cited its "longstanding safety record." Oil of oregano is especially popular among my clients for yeast infections. Try it for sinus infections, inhaled in a steam. It's often used topically or as a drop under the tongue, diluted it in a mild-flavored oil like olive oil. Don't take too much internally though.

Olive leaf extract is another all-around antimicrobial, and I know it sounds like we're getting ready to make salad dressing! Effective against both bacteria and fungi, it's especially useful for respiratory and GI bugs.

Colloidal silver is another extremely popular supplement for infections ranging from the most common cold and flu to the most dangerous bacteria like MRSA. It's the best of these three when you need something to take internally and work throughout your whole system against a bacterial infection. It is typically taken orally in drop form or as a spray for colds, sore throats, and sinus infections. It's safe as long as you follow the safety guidelines at www.silversafety.org.* Sovereign Silver and Silver Wings are excellent brands.

Your Shortcut Guide to Supplements

Basic daily supplements

- ∾ a smoothie with Green Vibrance from Vibrant Health

- ∾ a good multivitamin and (in winter) extra vitamin D

- ∾ essential fatty acids like Nordic Naturals Ultimate Omega

- ∾ probiotics such as Jarrow, Garden of Life, Renew Life

- ∾ magnesium such as Natural Calm

- ∾ N-acetylcysteine (NAC), 600 mg.

Immune support for when you're sick or feeling run down

- ∾ Source Naturals Wellness Formula or

- ∾ Gaia Herbs Quick Defense

- ∾ NAC 1200 mg, American ginseng, and/or using a neti pot**

Antimicrobials to work against bacteria, viruses, fungi

- ∾ colloidal silver, olive leaf, and/or oregano oil

---

*The "blue man" in the news recently was trying to make colloidal silver at home (bad idea) and consuming his home brew (which was *not* colloidal silver) by the glassful for years (*really* bad idea). "Anything in excess has consequences. Common substances like table salt and aspirin are harmless with normal use, but excessive intake can become toxic and even life-threatening. With normal responsible usage, silver supplements are entirely harmless to humans." —Jeffrey Blumer, MD, PhD; former director of the Center for Drug Research and of the Greater Cleveland Poison Control Center, quoted on www.silversafety.org.

**Here's how to tell which one you need. If you feel susceptible because you are overworked, underslept, and exhausted, take American ginseng. If you're mostly fine but still getting sick, take NAC. If you're constantly exposed to sick people (in a classroom, on the subway) use a neti pot daily. Or use all of the above!

Herbs for Your Cough: Many Uses, Many Forms

And now for the herbs, these wonderful plants used to heal humanity since time immemorial. Plants can be used to combat fungi, bacteria, and viruses. Ever wonder why? It's because they have to fight off the same types of invaders!

You'll find a bewildering array of herbs in your local health food store. How to decide which ones are best for your cough? Here are a couple of questions to consider:

- What kind of cough do I have?
  - dry or productive (mucusy)
  - tickly, spasmodic, or croupy, or
  - a cough that lingers after a cold or flu.
- How would I like to use my herbs?
  - brew a hot cup of herb tea
  - use an essential oil in a vaporizer or massage, or
  - keep it simple, take an herbal blend in a tablet.
- Would I rather save time (buy pre-made blends) or save my money (make things from scratch)?

Are the choices making your head swim? If so, just swim on over to page 68 where I share a few of my favorite things. I hope you'll have such a good experience that you'll come back to this chapter and delve into the "green world" of medicinal plants. If you're already a health food store aficionado, you will appreciate the details in this chapter.

How will you use them—and who will you use them for?

You may want to avoid the more bitter-tasting herbs, especially for your children who will want the milder, sweeter herbs. **Goldenseal** is a powerful antimicrobial, but the bitter taste of this golden powder will make kids go "yuck." Herbs are generally safe for kids, but you do need to consider the taste!

Sweet herbs can be just as powerful: **elderberry**, for example, makes a delicious berry-flavored syrup that's effective against colds and flu.

Star anise makes a licorice-flavored tea reminiscent of Chinese cuisine; did you know that the active ingredient in Tamiflu was originally extracted and synthesized from star anise?

As for convenience, you may need a tickle-suppressing herb to have on hand for that cough that tries to erupt right in the middle of a big meeting at work or that's keeping your family awake at night. It's not convenient to boil up a pot of herb tea then, but you could keep a bag of herbal lozenges handy. Read on!

Save your money or save your time

As we consider the best herbs for different types of cough, we'll also mention different ways to use them, from the most convenient (buying them premixed in a blend) to the most natural (growing your own in a backyard garden or windowsill pot). The most convenient forms are usually the most expensive. If you're a working mom, you may often find that you're paying more for convenience because you just don't have time to make things at home. And when you're buying herbal supplements, the best quality herbs are also the most expensive, but they are worth it. The precious medicinal ingredients need to be carefully conserved during processing. If you try to save money with cut-rate herbs, you may be wasting your money on ineffective products.

Buying bulk herbs and mixing up your own teas can be a good compromise. Find a natural food store with jars of bulk herbs so you can try just a little bit of each one until you find a few that you and your family like and that also work for you. It takes some time at first, but once you get the hang of it, brewing up a cup of herb tea is easy and buying the herbs in bulk is more economical than teabags.

Dry throat, tickly cough

Let's start with that dry throat that causes your tickly cough. **Slippery elm** will soothe and moisten your throat, stopping the cough. It's extracted from the inner bark of the tree, so it's not something you'll be growing on your windowsill. Fortunately it's easily available in lozenge form: Two Trees, for example, combine slippery elm and a little maple syrup sweetener in a delicious lozenge.

Or you can get it as a tea: Throat Coat by Traditional Medicinals features slippery elm plus other soothing herbs like **marshmallow root** and other cough-stopping herbs like **wild cherry bark** and **licorice** which also provides a lovely sweet flavor. (Licorice is not recommended for babies and small children, nor for people on certain medications listed in the Safety section at the end of this chapter. That's why Traditional Medicinals makes a "Just For Kids" version of Throat Coat, without the licorice.)

If you want to get slippery elm as close to the source as possible, you can buy the powder in bulk to make tea. This pleasant-tasting powder is mild-flavored, even a little sweet. It's traditionally made by stirring a tablespoonful into a cup of boiling water. Honey, cinnamon, or other sweet spices can be used to flavor it. By the way, it will keep working all the way down your digestive system to soothe and heal the mucous membranes. Holistic physicians recommend it for irritable bowel syndrome.

Herbal cough drops
There are many other herbs that work for tickly coughs, not by slippery-coating the throat but by opening up the airways. To have them handy for that cough that strikes in the middle of a meeting or worship service, carry **herbal cough drops** with you. Ricola includes many of the best herbs for coughs and it's easily available in drugstores as well as health food stores. (This brand contains sugar or artificial sweeteners, which we do not recommend; it's listed here first only because it's the most widely available.)

Olbas focuses on the essential oils of menthol, eucalyptus, juniper, wintergreen, and clove, while Vogel's Pine cough drops have menthol and pine oils, sweetened with honey and pear extract. All three of these brands come from Switzerland, which has a long tradition of herbal health care.

Propolis lozenges provide the protective benefits of this remarkable substance used by bees to keep their hives sterile. It's a sticky resin exuded by trees to protect their buds against bacteria and fungus; bees gather it and use it in the hive as an antifungal, antibacterial, and anti-viral. Anti everything! and it will work for you too, in lozenges or in Gaia Herbs' Echinacea Goldenseal Propolis Throat Spray. My clients who cough because of a mold allergy report that propolis can be put into a special diffuser or vaporizer to clear a living space of mold, germs and pollution, just as it does in the hive.

Elderberry: the herb treasured by our elders from ancient times
Everyone in the family can enjoy **elderberry syrup,** which has been traditionally used for colds, coughs, and flu. Recent research has shown it is effective against the flu virus and potential superbugs. Just to be clear, elderberry helps to stop coughs by stopping the underlying infection. Your body is creating the cough for a reason, so you don't want to use a cough suppressant while the infection rages on.

Herbs can vary widely in quality and effectiveness, so buy a reputable brand. My personal favorite national brand is Gaia Herbs, which makes elderberry as a syrup as well as capsules. (Diabetics should use capsules because elderberry syrup is too sweet for them.) Sambucus by Nature's Way is another well-known national brand, in both syrup and tablet form; its tablets dissolve nicely in the mouth. I like to shop local, and an excellent local brand here in New England is Maine Medicinals, which blends elderberry syrup with other immune-supporting herbs.

Elderberry syrup is a great example of something you can make yourself. Even though it's easily available in stores, you may find it satisfying to brew up something healing for your family, and with your loving touch you can add the power of your own healing intention to the inherent power of the herb. This beautiful shrub bears large clusters of small dark purple berries in the fall. You can grow it in your backyard (and attract lots of birds) or find it growing wild throughout most of the United States.

Don't eat raw elderberries, as they can make you sick if not fully ripe. They are safe to eat when cooked: mash with an equal volume of grapes or other sweet fruit, cover with water, bring to a boil, and cook down to make your own elderberry syrup.

The cough syrup that works best for me: Planetary Formulas' Loquat Respiratory Syrup, which uses the Japanese herb **loquat leaf** for its ability to loosen mucus in the chest and reduce inflammation in the airways. It also has the Chinese herb **fritillary** to loosen thick, sticky phlegm and soothe the throat.

By the way, Planetary Formulas is an excellent brand combining the best of Eastern and Western herbs: their Echinacea-Yin Chiao formula blends our well-known immune herb with **Yin Chiao,** the cold and flu formula used for hundreds of years in Traditional Chinese Medicine.

Antispasmodic herbs for when you can't stop coughing

How about a spasmodic cough? You know when you start coughing and you just can't stop? Some of the herbs for coughing work specifically as antispasmodics. **Butterbur** is top of the list because it's also good for allergies (worked as well as Flonase in one study, as well as Allegra in another). So if your cough is allergy-related, butterbur is your best bet.

If you like to grow your own herbs, **catnip** is easy. It will take over your garden if you're not careful, and the neighborhood cats will have a field day with it. It may have a calming effect on your moods as well as your coughs, and it has a mucilage effect like slippery elm to calm a tickly cough. Your silvery-grey mound of a catnip plant will produce plenty of spikes of tiny purple flowers, which you gather to make catnip tea. Infuse the flowers by boiling water and taking it off the heat for a minute before adding the catnip flowers to let them steep. Strain out the flowers when the tea is cool enough to drink.

Natural decongestants and expectorants

Breaking up congestion that's rattling around in your lungs or stuffing up your nose might be your top priority for an herbal remedy. Herbs like **thyme** and **wild ivy** work well, for example in Bronchial Soothe by Enzymatic Therapy, another of my favorite brands. You can also use it for spasmodic coughs.

Another approach to thin mucus: N-acetylcysteine or NAC, one of those remarkable substances that helps a wide variety of ills. It's the active ingredient in the prescription drug Mucomyst: basically NAC in aerosolized form, Mucomyst breaks up congestion right away. NAC as a supplement takes longer to work (results usually noticeable within an hour) and will break up excess mucus anywhere in the body. Used for just a few days, 1200 mg a day is a safe and appropriate amount (a 600 mg capsule twice a day).

You can also use **enzymes** to break up mucus, as in the product Mucostop. While it's labeled as a nasal and sinus decongestant, experience shows that it also works for mucus in your lungs. Another combination of enzymes, Wobenzym, was shown in a research study to relieve symptoms of chronic obstructive bronchitis.

If your mucus is caused by postnasal drip, use Xlear (see p. 44) to dry up nasal secretions and safely fight germs.

Once you've loosened the mucus, you'll want an expectorant to help get it out: try Olbas Cough Syrup or a steam with eucalyptus oil.

Lingering cough and all-around good cough formulas

For that cough that just won't go away, or for times when you just can't decide what you need: Old Indian Wild Cherry Bark by Planetary Formulas includes nearly all the herbs we've mentioned, plus the Chinese herbs **fritillary** and **platycodon**. The children's version is not quite as strong, because it reduces the less-pleasant-tasting antiviral herbs, but that means it's also better tasting.

Another great all-purpose cough formula: Gaia's Bronchial Wellness (syrup or tea), and remember their Quick Defense as an all-around immune support when you're sick.

Two more remarkable natural healers

There are almost too many wonderful plant-based substances for healing; it's hard to choose. Feeling overwhelmed? You only need a couple of things that work for you and then you'll have friends for life. For now, have fun trying out different products.

Here are two more of my favorites because they have such a wide range of benefits, included for my health-food-store-aficionado friends:

- ᴄ Umcka products, in a wide array of syrups and chewables in different flavors, feature **pelargonium**, an herb that can speed healing of acute bronchitis and all the "friends" that come with it (cough, fever, headache, runny nose, mucus in the chest, fatigue).
- ᴄ **Medicinal mushrooms** like cordyceps and reishi to strengthen the immune system. Breathe by Host Defense is a great brand.

Your own herb garden: back yard or windowsill

We've talked about single herbs and pre-made blends you can buy as capsules, teabags or loose dried herbs. What about growing your own, or finding them in the woods nearby? Of the several dozen herbs that can potentially help a cough, chances are you can grow at least one of them in your climate, and that could be the best one for you. Plants have life-energy, known as *prana* or *chi* in the East. A living plant, grown or harvested with your own loving touch, will carry special healing energy for you and your family.

Sage, rosemary, thyme, and **peppermint** can be grown as windowsill herbs. (I have found that a small EarthBox is worth the investment as a windowsill planter because of the size and vigor of the plants it produces. It has a reservoir of water in the bottom, making it nearly impossible to kill the plants by forgetting to water them, as I can attest from personal experience.) The leaves of these plants can be used fresh or dried to make herb tea, although they would taste odd if blended together! Actually sage, rosemary, and thyme make a savory, fragrant blend reminiscent of turkey stuffing. Peppermint can be used to flavor hot tea or a cool drink.

Natural decongestants with essential oils

Certain **essential oils** work quickly to break up congestion: eucalyptus, peppermint, wintergreen, juniper, and oils from the cedar-balsam-spruce group. Use an Olbas inhaler (convenient to carry around), Olbas Oil (more concentrated and has more oils in the formula) or the old favorite, Vicks Vaporub. Essential oils are the reason why Vicks works!

Or experiment with buying the pure oils. They are quite economical because you only need a few drops in a bath, a steam, or a chest rub (see page 47). There are no side effects since you'll be using them externally. You can easily make your own custom-blended Vicks-type formula.

Pine, cedar, spruce: Essential oils from the aromatic needles of these trees make a wonderful steam to open up the airway passages. They will also make you feel as peaceful as if you were walking in a pine forest! I'm going to take a side trip here and recommend one of the all-time favorite products in my former health food store: Queen Helene Batherapy bath salts with pine essential oil will open your sinuses with steam and the essential oil, plus relax you at the same time.

Rosemary and lavender oils: These oils are powerful decongestants with no side effects. Try rubbing a few drops of both rosemary and lavender oils on the chest and back (diluted in a carrier oil like almond, sesame or olive oil). Or pour a drop or two onto a tissue and place it near your pillow. You can also mix the lavender and rosemary with a drop of almond oil, rub it on the palms of your hands and gently place some under your nostrils. Added bonus: they smell wonderful … Ahhh!

Camphor-menthol-eucalyptus rubs like Vicks can antidote homeopathic remedies (render them ineffective). So if you decide to use the natural medicines described in the next chapter, best not to use Vicks. Rosemary and lavender work as well and will not antidote remedies.

Here are other essential oils you might try: **tea tree oil**, also known as melaleuca, is a powerful antimicrobial and decongestant. It may be the strongest oil medicinally but it also has a strong odor! You could mix it with a fragrant essential oils: frankincense and myrrh, lemon, eucalyptus, thyme, and nutmeg have all been used as natural decongestants and/or antibiotics. Look for a health food store with testers of essential oils so you can pick one that appeals to you. Keep it simple: from this long list, you are bound to find a fragrance that appeals to you.

Essential oils are very concentrated; start with just a drop at a time. In Europe essential oils are taken internally, but in the U.S. we commonly hear that they are toxic taken internally. That's because Americans tend to believe that if something is good, more is better! If you can restrain yourself to just one drop of an essential oil, it's usually fine to take it internally. When you apply it externally, dilute it with a carrier oil such as coconut, almond, sesame or olive oil, so that it's not too strong for your skin.

Safety considerations for herbs

Just because something is natural doesn't mean it's always safe. Herbs are generally known to be safe, because they have stood the test of time: if they were toxic, our great-grandmother herbalists would have figured that out by now. But they knew to use herbs in moderation; any substance with a powerful medicinal effect can be toxic if you take too much.

Just to put these safety warnings in perspective, few medicinal herbs cause as many side effects as our most widely used herb, an herb that can cause insomnia, nervousness and restlessness, stomach upset, nausea and vomiting, increased heart and breathing rate, headache, anxiety, agitation, ringing in the ears, and irregular heartbeats, plus — in the long term — may contribute to osteoporosis and heart disease. Millions of Americans consume this herb (coffee!) daily, knowing they can simply reduce or stop if they feel these side effects. If you're comfortable drinking coffee, you can feel comfortable using our recommended herbs, because you already know how to moderate your consumption. Here are some specific cautions, though:

Herbs while pregnant: Check with a health care professional trained in herbal medicine and in Dr. Aviva Romm's *The Natural Pregnancy Book.*

Herbs while nursing: Avoid large amounts of energizing or endocrine-affecting herbs such as ginseng. Our strong antimicrobials may make your milk taste unpleasant. Your baby will let you know if this is a problem!

Herbs in childhood: In general, as soon as children can eat adult foods, they can safely use adult herbs, although they may not like the taste. Reduce amounts proportionately by bodyweight.

Herbs for the elderly: Start with smaller quantities for the frail elderly to make sure they can tolerate medicinal herbs comfortably. Be aware of herb-drug interactions, keeping in mind that little research has been done in this area and the information you will find online may be based on just a few incidents. Check https://www.standardprocess.com/MediHerb-Document-Library/Catalog-Files/herb-drug-interaction-chart.pdf

Catnip: avoid if on sedative medication (consider using calming herbs instead of the sedative medication, in the long run). Also do not use if you are on lithium, because it has a diuretic effect and therefore can affect your lithium levels.

Colloidal silver: safe, as is ionic silver, however the inexpensive substitutes could be dangerous. See www.silversafety.org to learn how to distinguish among the types of silver and how to calculate a safe upper limit based on only 25% of the EPA's recommended daily limit.

Elderberry: if you decide to make your own elderberry syrup, remember that the berries need to be cooked, not eaten raw.

Licorice: not advisable for children. Use cautiously for anyone with high blood pressure, especially those on ACE inhibitors (diuretics are safe) or Cilostazol.

Olive leaf extract: high doses are used to reduce high blood pressure so it may not be safe for those with low blood pressure.

Thyme: be cautious if on blood thinners as it might enhance their effect. (We are talking about medicinal amounts here. A sprinkle of thyme used in cooking is safe.)

Liquid herbs: Read the label carefully because some herbal preparations are more concentrated than others. If you switch brands, a stronger one could be unpleasant tasting and possibly unsafe.

Topical applications: Vicks VapoRub and other topical ointments should not be rubbed in or near the nose as they can be inhaled into the lungs and, long term, can damage the lungs. Also, as a rare but possible danger with essential oils, they can catch fire if heated too hot over a candle, or if clothing or towels with essential oils on them are in a hot dryer.

Your Shortcut Guide to Herbs for Coughs

All-around great cough syrups for any kind of cough

- ∾ Planetary Formulas Old Indian or Loquat Respiratory Syrup

All-around immune support while you have a cough

- ∾ Elderberry syrup such as Sambucus by Nature's Way
- ∾ Umcka products
- ∾ Gaia Quick Defense

Dry throat, tickly cough

- ∾ Throat Coat Tea by Traditional Medicinals
- ∾ Two Trees lozenges with slippery elm
- ∾ Olbas, Vogel or Ricola herbal lozenges

Spasmodic cough

- ∾ Gaia's Bronchial Wellness
- ∾ Butterbur (especially if also having allergies)

Productive cough, to thin the mucus and help expectorate

- ∾ Bronchial Soothe by Enzymatic Therapy
- ∾ NAC (n-acetylcysteine), Mucostop or Wobenzyme
- ∾ Olbas Cough Syrup to help expectorate
- ∾ Xlear nasal spray to stop post-nasal drip

Essential oils to inhale or apply topically

- ∾ Vicks VapoRub, Olbas Oil

In the next chapter we'll learn about a form of medicine that I like to think of as the ultimate mind-body medicine, because it can be so effective at helping with stress at the same time that it addresses physical conditions.

๛ SIX ๛

Homeopathy: European Medicine

Dr. Gus calls homeopathy "European medicine" because he says his European colleagues are "using homeopathy to great advantage." When he goes to international pulmonology conferences, he hears that his fellow physicians from Germany, France and other European countries are using homeopathy effectively for coughs and he wanted to write this book, in part, to introduce Americans to homeopathy for coughs.

Can you imagine a form of medicine that comes on sweet little pellets that your kids love to take and so inexpensive that you can afford to buy several small tubes for home and purse? These humble medicines are hiding in plain sight in your health food store and pharmacy. You've probably never noticed them, and you've probably never heard of them (because their makers can't afford million-dollar ads on TV) ... until now. Welcome to the world of homeopathy.

Homeopathy has other advantages. It's nontoxic and not habit-forming; in fact as you take the remedies* over time, you should need them less and less. They often restore health in other ways than just stopping a cough. They can bring back your normal energy and mood. You might see a child who becomes whiny or cranky when she's sick return to her normal cheerful and cooperative self.

---

*Homeopathics are commonly called remedies because they have such a long history of being used in home care. The FDA categorizes them as over-the-counter medicines. In this book the terms "homeopathic medicines" and "homeopathic remedies" are used interchangeably.

Best of all, if your child wakes with a fever and cough, and it looks like you'll have to stay home from work to take her to the pediatrician, homeopathy can sometimes change her symptoms within the hour. Herbs and vitamins are wonderful and certainly important to support a healthy immune system—important to keep her from getting sick in the first place—but when she's already sick, it's too late for echinacea or vitamin C to get her well on the spot.

Any downside? It can take a little time to find the remedy that works best for you or your child, and a little more time to get the hang of how often to take it and when to stop. That's one reason why homeopathy is not included in our healthcare system: physicians don't have enough time with a patient.

Busy physicians and busy parents can skip the rest of this chapter and go straight to the "shortcut guide" on page 86. My fellow nurses will appreciate the information in this chapter, though, because we are trained to look at the whole person—mental, emotional, behavioral and social as well as physical. Parents who take the time with this chapter can find remedies for your children that will help support their growth and development and break the downward spiral of repeated antibiotics as well as treating their current cough or cold or flu.

To find the best remedy for your specific type of cough, you'll need to notice details like what triggers the cough (talking? going out in cold air?), what the mucus is like (if any), and how your moods have changed. It will require paying attention to your symptoms, a lost art in our fast-paced modern lifestyle.

Noting your specific symptoms is like getting fitted for a custom-tailored suit. It's worth it, because once you find a remedy that really nails your cough symptoms, it's likely to work for all your future coughs, because people tend to get sick in the same way. Your symptoms will be different from your family members', perhaps, but consistent for you. Not only that, your cough remedy might also well work for colds, flus and other acute illnesses.

But you're sick right now, and you don't have time to do a Sherlock

Holmes investigation of your cough symptoms. Here's the shortcut: a **combination remedy.** In homeopathy, this term refers to a handful of some common cough remedies packaged together by a particular brand, with each company choosing a different set of favorite remedies out of the dozens of possible cough remedies. If you're lucky, your best remedy is included in the first combination you try, and it works like a charm. Less lucky, the combination includes a pretty-good remedy for you and helps you get by. Worst-case scenario, you just spent less than $20 on a product which lasts for years and just might work for someone else in the family.

Let's take a closer look at these combination remedies, easily available in any health food store, many pharmacies, and online. All of them get a stunning 5 out of 5 (or very close to that) in online reviews by satisfied users.

Pharmacists' top recommended homeopathic cough product for children is **Hyland's Cough Syrup 4 Kids,** which includes four of the top cough remedies in a sugar and honey base. Hyland's also offers a cough formula in pellet form. Pellet combinations are more economical per dose and easier to carry around (no risk of leakage). Hyland's pellet formula blends three homeopathic remedies, two of which are different from those in the syrup. So if one product does not work, it's worth trying the other. Their **Cold 'n Cough Nighttime 4 Kids** has yet another combination of remedies, and by the way, it will work just as well for adults.

Chestal cough syrup, made by the top homeopathic pharmaceutical company in the world (Boiron), is the most widely distributed, so you're likely to find Chestal's bright orange label in your local drugstore. Like Hyland's, it contains both honey and sugar, however it lists honey first whereas Hyland's lists sugar first, so sugar-conscious consumers may prefer Chestal.

Another old favorite, **Cough & Bronchial Syrup,** is made by Boericke & Tafel, a homeopathic pharmaceutical company founded more than 150 years ago when homeopathy first came to America. (An advantage of homeopathy which we haven't mentioned yet: the medicines have stood the test of time.) This cough syrup is still around because it works so well, it is safe, and it contains some unusual remedies not found in any other combinations, so it's definitely worth checking out.

What if you try all of these products and none of them work? The most likely reason: out of dozens of possible cough remedies, you need one that's not in any of these blends. (Among all the products mentioned so far, only about 15 remedies are included.) Another possibility: you need stronger homeopathic remedies than are found in the blends, which are made in low potencies (i.e. mild strength) to accommodate sensitive people.

The strength of homeopathic remedies is indicated by the number after the name. "30c" is the most common strength for common ailments like coughs and colds. But look at the label of these blends. The ingredients are typically listed in a milder 3 or 6 potency. So please don't give up on homeopathy if the first one or two combination remedies don't help; your cough will just take a little more time to solve.

If you've found a combination product that works, why take the time and trouble to research your own special remedy, like the ones described in the rest of this chapter? One reason you already know: you can purchase your remedy separately in a higher (stronger) potency which means it will typically work faster.

There's more to homeopathy, though. Unlike conventional medications, which can cause side effects like drowsiness, a well-matching homeopathic remedy can bring side *benefits,* like improving your mood, energy and sense of well-being. A 30c potency is more likely to do that than the 3c or 6c in a combination formula.

I had a dramatic example of this: a 55-year-old tax accountant who came to see me for several problems including sinusitis. She liked doing everything naturally and had seen professional homeopaths for years, most recently one who had retired a year before. Already well educated in homeopathy, while waiting for her appointment with me she had found a combination sinus remedy, Sinusalia, which was working reasonably well.

Of the three ingredients in Sinusalia, I gave her the best-matching single remedy in a gentle 3c potency (as it appears in Sinusalia), as well as in the stronger 30c potency typically used for single remedies. I asked her to try each separately (the same remedy in a milder 3c potency and a stronger 30c potency) and compare their effectiveness.

Laura kept careful track of her symptoms—using a spreadsheet, of course! Interestingly, both products worked for her sinus congestion, however she liked the 30c version better because, she said, "I'm steady and even-keeled. My mood and energy are level." For a tax accountant heading into tax season, this was a big bonus! and for me, it was a great indication that higher potencies can help the mood.

Finding your best remedy: consider the cause

So let's consider how to find the best-matching homeopathic remedy for you and your cough. We'll need the details of your cough, such as whether it's a dry or productive (mucusy) cough, just as when you choose an OTC medication. We'll need even more details about what triggers it and what makes you feel better or worse. First, though, we'll consider something that conventional medicine does not usually take into account—and one reason why homeopathy can be so profoundly healing.

We'll look at the cause.

And we'll cast our net wide. Were you exposed to a cold wind? What kind? The cold dry blast from the blower on an airplane will require a different remedy from a cold wind comes up late in the afternoon, when kids have been running around and getting sweaty under their parkas, then suddenly chilled by the wind.

In homeopathy, we even look at emotional causes. Of course we recognize the role of viruses and bacteria, but we're more interested in susceptibility. If one person working in an office with ten other people comes down with the flu, why do two or three of his co-workers catch it and not the others? What can we do to help those two or three be as resistant as their fellow employees? Homeopaths look at many factors, with emotional stress being one of our specialties. Homeopathy has remedies for what we call "hearing bad news," for example. Did one employee just get a pink slip? Is another one worried about losing the mortgage on his home? Did one of them just find out her child is being bullied in school? Did another just get jilted in an email?

It's not just about the microbe

When one of my clients calls with a cold or cough, or if her child is sick, I get all the physical symptoms, and I also ask, "Is there anything that just happened that would have made you more susceptible to getting sick?" I explain that when we are stressed, we may "open the door" to the microbes that are all around us. If there is a *clear* stressor, I give that the highest priority in choosing a remedy, then I try to find a good match among the physical symptoms. Sometimes clients are unaware of any emotional trauma, but the physical symptoms lead me to suspect one.

For example, the mother of one of my little clients called because he had sore throat symptoms that led me to the remedy Lycopodium. Lycopodium is such a great remedy for victims of bullying, I asked her whether by any chance he had encountered bullying. People think I'm a mind-reader, but I'm not, I've just studied a lot of homeopathy! The mother confirmed that in fact she just found out he was being bullied, but she had not made the connection with his getting sick. I told her that Lycopodium not only was likely to help his sore throat, it was also—in my extensive experience with this remedy—apt to help him feel stronger inside and stand up to the bully, with the likely result that the bully would leave him alone.

In another example, I gave a remedy to a dear friend who had had a spasmodic cough for years since losing the love of her life to cancer. She only needed one dose of the remedy Ignatia—famous in homeopathy as the remedy for heartbreaks and other intense emotions—to silence the cough. She continued to take the remedy occasionally when the cough came back but only needed it rarely.

The mother of another little boy called when he had a cold and cough in June, an unusual time to get sick. I know that kids are under extra stress at the beginning and end of the school year, for various reasons, so I always ask about emotional causes. This seven-year-old had a best friend who lived close by; they waited for the school bus together and played together every day after school. Then one day toward the end of June, my young client walked to his friend's house, and no one was there. The family had moved and they thought they would spare both boys' feelings by not telling them ahead of time. So the boys didn't even have a chance to say goodbye.

We cannot underestimate the grief in the life of a child when losing a best friend like this. Boys are taught not to cry and teased as sissies if they do. With no way to express how they feel, their bodies find a way, "speaking" through the language of symptoms. The unshed tears of suppressed grief found expression through a typical symptom addressed by Natrum mur.,* our most common grief remedy: "albuminous" nasal discharge, like uncooked egg whites. Odd as this may sound to someone unfamiliar with homeopathy, as soon as the mother described her son's mucus, I knew to ask if there were a grief involved.

Natrum mur. immediately helped his cold, stopping his postnasal drip and therefore his cough. More importantly, it helped his mood as well. His mother had not thought to tell me that her son was unusually moody and withdrawn (typical Natrum mur. symptoms), but she reported that the remedy helped restore him to his usual sunny self. This is an example of the "side benefits" rather than "side effects" from homeopathic medicines. If his body had used a spasmodic cough to express how he was choking back his sobs, I would have given him Ignatia, another grief remedy, instead.

Possible causes: physical and emotional

So let's pause now to look at the remedies matching some common traumas, whether physical or emotional. Remember you would never give

---

*Homeopathic medicines have Latin names, which are sometimes so long that they are abbreviated, as in the case of Natrum muriaticum and Rhus toxicodendron. A period at the end of the name in this book indicates that it has been abbreviated; when you see it in the store, the name on the label will be much longer.

a remedy ONLY based on this list; it's just one important item in your symptom-gathering. Many times there is no known cause and we move ahead into the details of the symptoms. We'll talk about potency, dosage, and where to get the remedies later in this chapter.

- ∾ cold dry wind: **Causticum** or **Aconite** (the latter especially for kids running around and getting sweaty under their clothes)
- ∾ sudden fright such as a near-miss car accident: **Aconite**
- ∾ being treated unfairly or upset about injustice: **Causticum**
- ∾ separation anxiety in small children: **Pulsatilla**
- ∾ extreme anxiety about survival issues (money, job, home, health): **Arsenicum**
- ∾ being bullied: **Lycopodium**
- ∾ being humiliated, **Ignatia**
- ∾ hearing bad news: **Ignatia** or **Gelsemium**
- ∾ sudden grief: **Ignatia**
- ∾ long-term grief: **Natrum mur.**

A shift in temperament

Maybe there isn't a particular emotional *cause*, but you notice a shift in your *mood*, or your child's. Any mom can tell when her small child needs **Pulsatilla**: this child, normally sweet, affectionate and mild-tempered, becomes even more so when sick, wanting to climb on mom's lap and cuddle. She'll be so clingy, she won't let her mom leave the room, and she will cling to mom's legs like velcro when dropped off at daycare.

Pulsatilla is almost a universal remedy for minor infectious illnesses of childhood when the child has this kind of temperament—totally different from the grouchy "leave me alone" state that indicates the person may need **Bryonia**. (Some moms have been known to get into this state when sick!) Bryonia is called the "grouchy bear in a cave" remedy for good reason.

Other remedies for grouchy people include **Nux vomica** and **Hepar sulph.**, and they are similar in other ways. The irritable Nux-needing person is so chilly, he'll get in bed and pull the covers up to his chin, and if there's even a little crack that allows cold air in, he'll get really cranky. The Hepar sulph.-needing person is also chilly and irritable, although he's sensitive to both hot and cold as well as to being touched and to drafts of air.

Sometimes people become anxious rather than grouchy when they're sick. I mentioned that **Aconite** is the first remedy to think of when the person suddenly comes down with something after being frightened "to death." Well, honestly, that rarely happens. You're more likely to see the connection happen in reverse: the person gets sick, then gets anxious, sometimes even to the extent of believing they are going to die. You may think they're being melodramatic—"I'm not going to make it through the night!"—but they just need Aconite.

A more common remedy for very anxious people: **Arsenicum.** These people are likely to get totally self-absorbed in worrying about their own needs, wanting to make sure they have others around them organized to take care of all their survival issues. They need hot drinks for their sore throat, an ice pack for their headache, and reassurance that they won't lose their job if they miss another day of work because they are totally flattened from lack of energy. They will worry that if they miss work, they'll lose their job, then they won't be able to pay their mortgage, then they'll end up out on the street. Wait, how did we get from a simple cough to being homeless?

And what if the cough becomes a tic? Sometimes we see people, children especially, who develop a cough as a nervous habit. They may develop a constant throat-clearing or little cough that gets worse when they are stressed out. Kids like this may need Causticum, especially if the cough started after exposure to a cold wind or to an injustice ("it's just not *fair!*").

Or they may need the remedy **Cuprum.** People who need Cuprum are competitive, push themselves very hard in school and in sports, and are preoccupied with rules. They are sure to follow the rules themselves and they get anxious when others don't. ("Mom! You're supposed to put that in the *recycling* bin!" or "Mom! You're not supposed to park there!")

Teachers are likely to recognize at least one of these children in every class: They will "tell" when other kids do something "really bad" like cutting in line—not to be mean to others, but because the rules are so important to them. Their nervous-tic cough represents their inner conflict between holding themselves back by following the rules versus wanting to push ahead, to do their very best, to exert themselves *hard* in school and in sports.

Cuprum can be used for full-fledged coughs even when this personality trait is not present: Cuprum is used for any spasmodic condition in the body such as stomach cramps, hiccups or calf cramps, so the cough would be spasmodic. It's not the only remedy for spasmodic coughs (Ignatia is another one). If the cough comes on at 3 a.m., or if it's better when the person drinks cold water, it's likely to respond to Cuprum.

In homeopathy we prioritize the person's mental state and their mood shifts—IF these are dramatically different from usual; and an emotional trauma at the outset IF there was one. Of course, many times you'll just have physical symptoms to go on, and many remedies do not have a particular emotional state associated with them. And someone might well need a remedy we've just mentioned based on their *physical* symptoms, even if the associated *emotional* state is not present. Bottom line: prioritize any emotional clues, IF any. If not, go on to the physical symptoms.

If your cough is dry

So now let's consider the physical symptoms of the cough itself, beginning with the classic split between dry and "mucus-y" coughs. Dry coughs first:

Is it so painful to cough that you have to hold your chest? Take **Bryonia**, and keep this remedy in mind for the pain of bruised or fractured ribs as well. Bryonia is also likely to be used for a dry cough moving down into the chest. There's another way you can be sure Bryonia matches well: the person is very thirsty and likely to gulp down a lot of water at once. They may be thirsty because they feel their mouth is dry. "Bry drinks the ocean dry" is the rhyme that homeopathy students use to remember this symptom.

Phosphorus is another wonderful remedy for dry coughs that are on their way down into the chest from a cold. The Phosphorus cough is likely to be triggered by talking, laughing, or going out into the cold air. These are pretty common symptoms, though, so you are more likely to recognize the person needing Phosphorus by the temperament: even when she's sick, she's likely to look fine and have plenty of energy, especially when it comes to going out and doing something fun with her friends. Phosphorus is also my favorite medicine for coughs triggered by fumes, fragrances, household cleansers and other substances containing toxic chemicals.

Does the cough tickle in the throat-pit (the hollow between the collarbones?) Consider **Rhus tox.** or **Rumex**. If by chance the person also has fever blisters that look like poison ivy (little fluid-filled blisters), you can be sure Rhus tox. will help both symptoms.

Rumex is your other "tickle in the throat pit" cough remedy, although it also works well when the tickle is farther down where the trachea (windpipe) branches. You might feel as though you have a little tiny piece of something deeper in your chest, like a little sliver of paper that you desperately want to cough out, but you just can't, and it makes you crazy. Like Phosphorus, Rumex is good for a cough brought on by talking or going out into cold weather, so these people are especially likely to cover their mouth with a scarf in cold air.

Croupy coughs

Spongia is used when the tickling is so relentless, the person just can't stop coughing a dry, hard, barking cough which can even sound like sawing wood. The cough can be triggered by being over-excited, by taking a deep breath, or drinking cold drinks, and conversely relieved by drinking hot drinks. It's one of the best remedies for croup.

Sometimes the best way to find the best-matching remedy has to do with the person's position. If your child starts to cough as soon as she lies down in bed, think of **Drosera**. You'll need to be sure: is this a positional issue, or a time-of-day issue? When someone needs **Drosera**, though, the cough is triggered by lying down, not necessarily at night. You can tell by asking the mom whether the same thing happens if her child lies down for a nap. Drosera is one of the remedies for a whooping or croupy or barking cough (sounds like a seal), along with **Spongia** (for the cough that sounds like sawing wood).

Many remedies are associated with a certain time of day or night. **Aconite**, for example, is associated with waking at midnight, suddenly sick with a fever after feeling fine when going to bed. Someone needing **Arsenicum** is likely to be awake in the wee hours *after* midnight, restless and anxious, pacing around unable to sleep.

For croup, there are three remedies that work so well, it would be wise to have all of them on hand if your child is in the age range likely to get it. Use **Aconite** if you can catch it right in the beginning. Someone who needs Aconite is likely to go to bed feeling just fine, then wake up around midnight suddenly feeling very ill with really strong symptoms: a high fever, restlessness, and possibly a lot of anxiety about being sick. Or possibly your child was overly chilled the previous day. A dose or two of Aconite in the middle of the night, and your child may be better in the morning, because we tend to heal while we sleep.

But what if you're new to this and you don't have Aconite on hand? The cough may do what we call "progressing": moving to the next phase, with the next set of symptoms. The next stage of croup is likely to need **Spongia,** for the barking cough that sounds like sawing wood. Again, if you don't catch it in time it's likely to reach the more infectious and "mucus-y" **Hepar sulph.** stage. These three remedies are called the "classic croup triad" of Aconite–Spongia–Hepar sulph. Of course if your child can't breathe, you'll be heading to the ER first!

Note the body language

Kali carb. is distinguished by the person needing to lean forward with their elbows on their knees in order to cough. This is another "time of day" cough, or rather "time of night": someone needing Kali carb. will wake up around two to four in the morning with a racking cough.

Remember ipecac, the old-time remedy for nausea and vomiting? If so, it will be easy to remember the homeopathic remedy **Ipecac**: sufferers lean over and cough so hard they vomit, or feel like they are about to.

Productive (phlegmy or mucusy) coughs

Now on to the mucus. In homeopathy, we are fascinated by mucus. What color is it? Is it thick or thin? What part of the chest is it in? If people need **Causticum**, they may feel mucus on their larynx, which they try to cough up but can't get all the way out so they need to swallow it. Another huge hint for Causticum: "stress incontinence," a fancy term for leaking a bit of urine when you cough or sneeze. Also your throat may feel raw and sore "like someone scraped it with a vegetable peeler," as one of my clients described it.

If they need **Hepar sulph.**, you may hear the rattle of mucus in the middle of the chest behind the sternum (breastbone). People who need Hepar sulph. are very sensitive to both heat and cold, to drafts, to being bumped into … just about anything makes them grouchy.

If the cough has been going on for a while and the mucus has settled in the bottom of the lungs, try **Ant. tart.** (our rather unappetizing nickname for Antimonium tartaricum, the full name on the label). Not only is the mucus low in the lungs, the person needing Ant. tart. is too weak to cough it up and out, so it is especially useful for elderly people.

Mucus like uncooked egg whites (clear as water but thicker) means the person is likely to need **Nat. mur.**, the same remedy you met in the story of the little boy who missed his best friend.

Thick, sticky mucus anywhere in the body is likely to need **Kali bic.** (short for Kali bichromicum). It can be used for nasal discharge in long strings or plugs (the technical term for these is "boogers"), for postnasal drip, for mucus in the throat that's hard to hawk out, and for mucus blocking the sinuses or ears. On page 34 we talked about how to feel above and below your eyes to see if you have pain or tenderness. If you find pain in a small spot, a dime-sized spot, that's a good clue that Kali bic. will help. Research in Austria has documented its effectiveness in clearing mucus from the lungs of patients on ventilators.

Dr. Gus used Kali bichromicum for one of his patients, a 98-year-old woman who was being cared for at home by her husband following hospitalization for pneumonia. She had so much difficulty breathing that she required surgery to insert a tube into her throat. This tube was attached to a "vent" or ventilator, a piece of medical equipment that pushes air into the person's lungs. On the one hand, the vent was keeping her alive, for which she and her husband were grateful. But it meant that she could not speak or leave her bed, so her quality of life was not so good. And when people have a "trache" (tracheotomy, or breathing tube in their throat), mucus can build up in their lungs until they have the terrifying feeling of almost suffocating.

Her husband called Dr. Gus, begging for anything that might get her off the vent. Over the next six months they tried a diuretic, Mucomyst, nebulizers, and a $10,000 chest percussion vest, to no avail. Finally Dr. Gus suggested Kali bichromicum. Three days later a jubilant husband called to report: the remedy worked so well to reduce her mucus, she was now able to breathe on her own. She was finally able to leave the house during the day, and she was drinking champagne with her husband to celebrate!

Note that a $7.95 tube of a homeopathic remedy just saved the healthcare system tens of thousands of dollars. She no longer needed a ventilator machine or oxygen during the day, nor frequent visits from a visiting nurse or respiratory therapist to remove the mucus from her lungs, and her multiple medications were reduced. Even though monumental costs like this are usually covered by Medicare or insurance, all of us end up paying for them indirectly through taxes or insurance premiums.

The cost savings were not the most important factor, of course. If you could see the look of terror in the eyes of someone on a ventilator having difficulty breathing, you would agree that getting her life back was the most important result.

Finding and taking the remedies

I hope these dramatic stories have inspired you to try homeopathy! The special remedies described here are "hidden in plain sight" in your health food store, and a handy summary is in Appendix E. The combination remedies and cough syrups mentioned earlier are likely to be in your drugstore as well. Your neighborhood health food store is more likely to have a sales staff trained to answer questions about homeopathy.

Most often the store will have a plexiglas dispenser with several dozen remedies in light blue tubes a little smaller than lipstick tubes: the Boiron brand. They often will have another brand nearby in small white plastic bottles with red caps: the Hylands brand. A well-stocked store will have the Boericke & Tafel (B&T) brand. You can find all these brands and others online. The brand is less important than with herbs and vitamins, because the FDA categorizes homeopathic medicines as drugs and standardizes their manufacture. The brands differ when it comes to the combination remedies described in the beginning of the chapter, because each company chooses different homeopathic medicines for its blend.

For single remedies, most people will do well with the most common potency, 30c. People who are extremely sensitive may need the gentler 6c or 12c potency. (Higher numbers mean stronger medicine.) Two pellets dissolved in the mouth are enough for a dose. To make it stronger, take it *more often* rather than taking *more pellets*. Here's why.

Homeopathic medicines work by conveying information to your body's healing energy, reminding it how to be healthy. Each time you take a dose, the healing energy is reminded again. Imagine you want to learn a song. You would learn it better by having a couple of people sing it over and over ten times, rather than by listening to ten people sing it just a couple of times. Repetition is key. So doubling the number of pellets in a dose doesn't double the strength.

As for how often, the label on the tube may say to take it three times a day, but that's a generic suggestion. Better to adapt the frequency to your own circumstances by understanding how the remedies work. You want to take enough to get the ball rolling, and as soon as healing is underway, let the body's own healing powers take over. You're trying to nudge it in the right direction with each dose, and as soon as it starts moving in the right direction on its own, leave it alone.

It's especially obvious with kids when the remedy kicks in. Their appetite comes back, they get color back in their faces, and they're interested in their favorite games or shows again. You can feel it in yourself when pain subsides or drippiness starts to dry up.

Since we're focused on coughing here, you can use the cough itself as a benchmark for how often to give the remedy. Try taking the remedy each time you cough (but no more than once every couple of hours). As the remedy works, you won't need it as often and you will naturally slow down.

What if you're not getting better? Consider how sure you are of your remedy choice. If you were torn between two remedies, I would try one consistently for a day but if you're no better the next morning, try the other one. We heal while we sleep, so we often find we've turned the corner on an acute illness when we wake up the next morning.

On the other hand, if the main problem is that the symptoms are extremely powerful, try making the remedy stronger by putting it in water: dissolve two pellets in half a cup of water (4 oz. or 125 ml), crush if necessary or stir to dissolve, stir really well and keep sipping on it. Putting the remedy in a small amount of water seems to deliver the information more efficiently via the mucous membranes inside your mouth.

For a baby, to avoid having the baby inhale a pellet, either crush the pellet and put a little powder inside the baby's mouth, or dissolve it in a little water and dab it on lips, temples or the inside of the wrist.

What if your symptoms are different the next day but you still feel sick? Congratulations, you did a great job! You moved your cough, cold or flu along to the next stage, requiring a different remedy. Most people are sick for two or three weeks with a cold or flu, going through different stages from watery mucus to thick dry mucus at the end, or from a head cold to mucus in the mid-chest to trying to cough it up from the base of the lungs at the end. With homeopathic remedies, you could go through the stages in just three days and feel totally better by the fourth day. Pat yourself on the back!

Getting the hang of this—noticing when to repeat a remedy

❧ SEVEN ❦

Body, Mind and Spirit:
Natural Therapies

Breath and spirit are connected in the language and beliefs of cultures around the world. Our own words "inspiration" and "aspiration" refer to breathing in and are also connected to "spirit." "Respiration" contains the same root, as does "expiration" for the moment when we breathe our last, when we "give up the ghost." The Holy Ghost of the Christian Trinity, also called the Holy Spirit, is *pneuma* in the Greek of the New Testament. Also meaning "breath" or "lung," *pneuma* is the root of "pneumonia" and other lung-related medical terms.

Meanwhile the Hebrew *ruach* carries the same range of meanings: spirit or breath. In India, *pranayama* refers to the breathing exercises of yoga: breathing in *prana,* the universal life-force, brings us closer to Spirit. *Chi* or *qi*, the life force in Traditional Chinese Medicine, originally meant breath or air. To a *chi gung* practitioner, coughing can actually be beneficial, a form of internal massage stimulating a healthy flow of *chi* among our three *dan tiens* (energy centers).

Breathing exists at the threshold between our physical body and our conscious awareness. We all know that when we feel tense, our chest tightens and our breathing becomes shallow. Remarkably, the opposite is also true. If we notice we are feeling tense, we can choose to take a few long deep breaths to relax. We have just used our physical body to change our emotional state. (Breathing in a relaxing essential oil at the same time can be even more stress-reducing; my own favorite is a pine oil that brings hints of the deep pine woods.)

In this chapter we will look at things we can do with our mind and body to help heal a cough, beginning with the powerful Buteyko breathing method.

Buteyko: effortless breathing

"You just tell them to stop coughing?" a pulmonologist asked incredulously. "And they can *do* it?" A Buteyko breathing educator was explaining this revolutionary method of treating asthma and other chronic coughs to her fellow staff members at Boston Medical Center. Hadas Golan, a dynamic and ebullient Israeli speech pathologist, was eager to explain her success with the pulmonologists' patients.

When there is a mismatch between the severity of the symptoms and the lung function test, pulmonologists sometimes suspect that the problem is caused by the upper airways and diagnose "vocal cord dysfunction." They then refer the patient to a speech pathologist trained to treat vocal cord dysfunction. Fortunately the speech pathologist in the otolaryngology department at Boston Medical Center was also trained in the Buteyko method. As the pulmonologists began hearing back from their patients about remarkable improvements, they would refer more and more of their patients to Golan.

"Every medical student learns the physiological principles behind the method," Golan explains. "Conventional doctors are not trained to assess or treat breathing behaviors. They focus on the use of medications and procedures to treat symptoms. The Buteyko method addresses the root causes of these symptoms—a physiological imbalance. The focus of breathing retraining is to correct the breathing habits that cause or aggravate the problem. Once physiologically normal breathing is restored, symptoms improve, and less medication is required."

The principles behind the Buteyko method are both deceptively simple and also counter-intuitive. Breathing in brings in life-giving oxygen (O_2); breathing out rids the body of carbon dioxide (CO_2), the toxic waste product of metabolism. We cannot live for even a few minutes without oxygen; if we try to hold our breath, our oxygen levels plummet until finally the brain, starved of oxygen, makes us gasp for air. Right?

Actually, no. That's what we learned in high school biology, but the reality is not as simple as "oxygen = good, CO_2 = bad, and lack of oxygen drives the urge to breathe." As medical students learn, carbon dioxide isn't all bad—for example, without enough CO_2, the blood does not release oxygen into the tissues—and in fact it is the *buildup of CO_2* that drives the urge to breathe. The real problem underlying many chronic breathing-related diseases is not lack of oxygen but hyperventilation driving out too much CO_2. This disrupts the balance between the O_2 and CO_2 in the lungs and blood, affecting pH regulation and other vital bodily functions, and in severe cases may cause system-wide physiological crisis.

The Buteyko method, developed by a Russian physician in the 1950s, is based on this simple concept. We are taught that deep breathing is healthiest, but actually it drives out too much CO_2 and then we fail to breathe properly. Asthmatics and people with other illnesses (diabetes, heart disease, anxiety) tend to breathe two to three times more air than the norm and are chronically low in CO_2. Deep breathing is really only appropriate for exercise, while for daily life we need to breathe as babies do: relaxed, through the nose, and from the diaphragm. You can see babies' abdomens rise and fall slightly as they breathe.

Babies, of course, are totally relaxed; they spend most of their time sleeping! But when we are stressed, the fight-or-flight response triggers a number of changes in our bodies, preparing to save us from the saber-tooth tiger that never shows up in our sedentary world. One of the basic changes with the fight-or-flight response is that breathing increases, in case we need to run away from the tiger, but of course in our modern world we can't cope by running away. You may feel that your boss is like a saber-tooth tiger, but as long as you're working at a computer, that physical fight-or-flight response doesn't help!

In our wired, fast-paced, stressed-out world, we live in such a constant state of overbreathing that it becomes a habit we're not even aware of. Buteyko coined a term for this: "hidden hyperventilation." People typically don't recognize the signs that they are overbreathing:

- breathing with the mouth open,
- visible movement in the upper chest or abdomen,
- audible breathing,
- snoring, or
- sighing and yawning a lot.

But it all adds up because we are breathing 20,000 to 30,000 times a day. In fact people are sure they are *not* overbreathing, because they *feel* short of oxygen, until they try this more relaxed and shallow method and find they have more oxygen.

The Relaxed Breathing exercise

You can use the Buteyko method when you have an acute cough, but first let's learn some basic Buteyko breathing by practicing its Relaxed Breathing exercise:

- Sit in a tall, comfortable posture.
- Fully relax the muscles by shrugging your shoulders so they rest on your rib cage instead of being tensed up around your neck.
- Allow your stomach to soften.
- Breathe through your nose if possible.
- Allow the breathing to happen without you doing anything.

The body will "breathe itself" and you will notice that there is less and less movement in the upper chest and abdomen. You are breathing from a smaller "container," and you feel like you are not breathing as much as you are used to, but actually you are breathing very efficiently.

Remember to always breathe through your nose, not just while inhaling, to keep the airway moist. Nose-breathing benefits anyone with a cough, because it moistens and sterilizes the airway and reduces the irritation that causes coughing. A moister airway keeps the mucus thin; thicker mucus makes for harder coughing, which can irritate the airway.

Then it becomes harder to clear the mucus … so you instinctively cough … creating a vicious cycle.

Of course many people with coughs also have stuffed-up noses (a good time for a neti pot or saline rinse as described on p. 44-45). The Buteyko method will gradually take care of the stuffiness, making nose-breathing possible, but the transition is best supervised by a professional if you have chronic congestion.

See the diagram on the cough cycle, on the next page. (Note to physicians: "CO_2 pressure drops" refers to CO_2 in the alveoli, not in the blood.)

Cough medications work to thin or dry out the mucus, suppress/numb the irritation sensation, or force the airways open, but they don't address the root cause and sometimes make it worse in the long run. Buteyko addresses the overbreathing, restores gentle nasal breathing, and thus addresses the root cause and reverses the cycle.

So here is how to use the Buteyko principles for an acute cough. The idea is to substitute a swallow of water for a cough, because the swallow is less traumatic to the tissues. The less you cough, the less irritated the vocal folds are, the less mucus they produce, then they can heal, so the less you have to cough. This way you can reverse the vicious cycle of coughing. It's very simple:

- Always keep a glass of water handy.
- When you feel the urge to cough, take a small sip.
- Swallow hard and try not to cough.
- If you absolutely have to cough after a few sips and swallows, do it like a silent throat clear, with your mouth closed.

Alternately, you can try to use the mini pause exercise:

- Comfortably breathe out through your nose.
- Pinch your nose.
- Pause your breath to the count of 5. Release.
- Gently nose breathe for 3-4 breaths.
- Repeat for 3-5 minutes or until the urge to cough is gone.

The Buteyko Explanation of the Cough Cycle

Airways cool and dry out

Traumatize vocal folds

More mucus is produced for protection and lubrication

More inhalation of irritants

Over-breathing / Cough

More irritation / Difficulty to breathe

Airways constrict

Smooth muscle constricts

CO_2 pressure drops

Blood vessels narrow

Heart has to pump harder

High blood pressure

The more you practice the Relaxed Breathing exercise and make gentle nasal breathing your new way of breathing, the quicker your irritated airway can recover. Many people believe they have to cough hard to clear their lungs, but gentle coughing is also effective. This way the airways will stay open, unlike the constricted airways in asthma, Golan explains. Phlegm will come up naturally without damaging the tissues of the throat or stressing the heart.

We will learn more about the Buteyko method for chronic coughs in chapter 11, "Chronic Hackers and the Art of Medicine."

Acupressure: like do-it-yourself acupuncture without the needles
Unlike acupuncture, acupressure is safe to practice on yourself at home. For the cough points in particular, since so many are on the back, you'll need a friend to press them for you. You may get even better results from a professional acupressure practitioner. (For a chronic cough, go to a professional acupuncturist for a protocol individually suited to your particular cough.)

There are many acupressure points for cough. The most effective points will vary depending on the individual but there are some points that are particularly common. There will almost always be tenderness at the point if it is effective. To manipulate a point, you do not have to use a tremendous amount of pressure. The goal is to stimulate the body to respond. If you use varying amounts of pressure (hold and release, hold and release) the body will stay more sensitive and you will get a better response.

When you look at the locations of these points, you may notice that a lot of them are on the chest and back. Their close proximity to the lungs helps reduce the cough. Almost all of these points will also help reduce the symptoms of a cold or flu. You can also do some *qi gong* self massage techniques to help circulate lymph in the neck, ears and throat.*

---

*These recommendations are from Dr. James Tin Yao So, founder of New England School of Acupuncture, via Jerry Kantor, LicAc, CCH, one of his first students; and from Jared West, L.Ac., the acupuncturist at Cleveland Clinic Ohio.

General acupressure points for cough
(see the diagrams on the following pages)

Don't worry about exact locations; just feel around in the general area until you find a tender or sore spot.

1. CV 17: the middle of the sternum between the nipples (at the level of the space below the fourth rib)

2. Lung 1: Put your arm out straight parallel to the floor and feel down from your shoulder to the deep pit below your collarbone and inside the shoulder.

3. Kidney 27: the depression below the collarbone, about 1.5″ away from the midline

4. The "Stop Cough" or "Stop Asthma" point just on either side of the spine at C7. (At the base of the neck, find the first "big bump" vertebra as you go down the spine.)

5. Bladder 12: about 1″ on either side of midline in the space between the second and third thoracic vertebrae. (The thoracic vertebrae are the larger bumps in your spine, as you proceed downward from the back of the head.)

6. Bladder 13: about 1″ on either side of midline at the third thoracic vertebra, just below Bladder 12.

7. Lung 5: just outside the large tendon in your elbow crease when you bend your elbow; Lung 5 is in the hollow formed by this tendon.

8. Lung 6: from Lung 5, go almost halfway to the wrist crease (where your hand begins) on the outside of your radius bone (the larger bone in the forearm), and find Lung 6 in a depression that you can feel.

Cough with phlegm

9. Stomach 40: Find the center point of your outer ankle bone and the crease behind your knee; halfway between these two points is the vertical dimension. Horizontally, find the outer edge of the tibia (main bone in the lower leg) and go ½″ further away from midline, at that halfway vertical point.

Cough with anxiety

10. Heart 6: about 1/2" above the wrist crease, between the large tendon at the base of the thumb and the tendon next to it.

Cough with head conditions (sinusitis, runny nose, headache)

11. Large Intestine 4: at the top of the mound formed on the back of your hand when you press the thumb and forefinger together.

Cough with fever

12. GV14: on the midline just above the first thoracic vertebra, which is just below the first "big bump" vertebra at the base of the neck as you go down the spine.

Acupressure for colds and lymphatic drainage

There are two acupressure techniques that Jared West commonly uses for the ears and throat. He has found both to be very effective at improving local circulation, lymphatic drainage and — because of their location — reducing the symptoms of the common cold.

1. Place the index finger behind the ear and the middle finger in front of the ear so that the fingers form a V. Then lightly rub the fingers on either side of the ear. The skin should start to feel warm but not irritated or uncomfortable at all. If becomes at all uncomfortable, use less pressure. Continue lightly rubbing for 30-60 seconds.

2. Place the thumb and index finger of the same hand on either side of the throat beginning just under the jaw bone. Using very light pressure slide them down the throat to the middle of the chest. Alternate hands using very minimal pressure. This will help the lymph move through the throat and stimulate acupressure points in the chest that govern breathing and immunity. It also feels good for a sore throat. Continue alternating hands for 60 seconds. Again, stop if this becomes uncomfortable particularly if you feel any dizziness during the exercise.

West has never actually seen someone become dizzy with the second exercise, but he says that too much pressure could do that, so be sure to use a light touch.

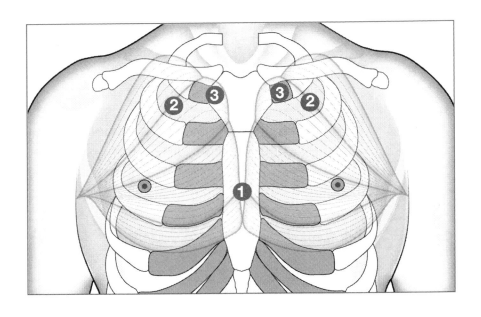

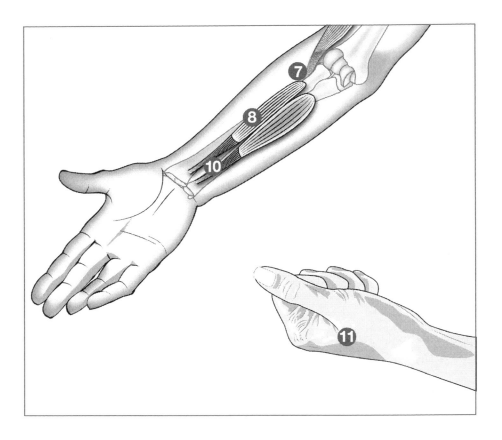

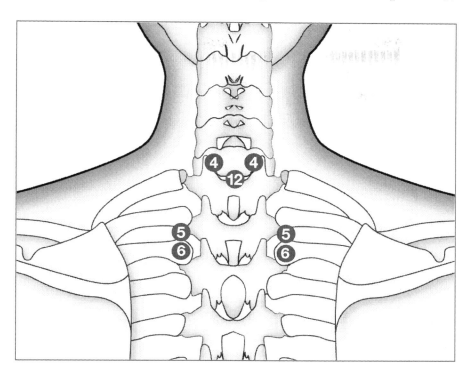

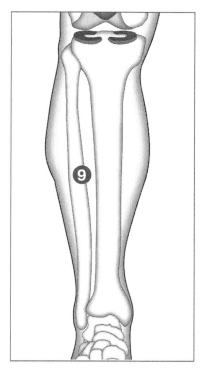

Fasting

Fasting (in its strictest form, avoiding all food and drink except water) has been used since ancient times for healing and spiritual renewal. Fasting is a natural way to let the body focus on healing, because digestion uses up so much energy. Even animals tend to hide away and avoid eating while sick in order to conserve their energy for healing.

Modern research has documented the effectiveness of fasting—and of its milder version, longterm calorie reduction—for preventing aging, supporting the immune system, and treating a wide range of conditions such as anxiety, high blood pressure, epilepsy and obesity. In a study in Ukraine, for example, a three-day course of fasting was effective for pre-asthma and bronchial asthma patients, plus they had fewer viral infections.

And in the study most closely related to our topic of acute coughs, rats who were not allowed to eat for 24 hours had less histamine release than their free-feeding buddies. What's so special about preventing histamine release? If you've ever taken an antihistamine, you know what misery histamines can cause in terms of a runny nose and itchy eyes. The lab technicians in this experiment actually counted how many times the little furballs sneezed and rubbed their noses with their tiny paws after being exposed to an allergen.

Dr. Gus cautions that patients with diabetes should not practice fasting without consulting a doctor (because it can cause a dangerous drop in blood sugar). It would be wise for anyone with a chronic disease to consult a doctor who understands the value of fasting.

We are including fasting in this chapter because Dr. Gus uses fasting and prayer to treat his own acute illnesses. Whether he wakes up with an upset stomach, sore throat, or the early stage of flu, Dr. Gus follows his morning prayer practice with a day of herbal teas and fruit juices, plus plenty of water. If at all possible, he also observes an electronics fast, keeping a silent and devout atmosphere by turning off his phone, iPad, and computer.

Dr. Gus admits that it's hard to go to work on the first day of a fast, when most people tend to feel weak and tired. But by the next day he usually feels fully recovered and extra-energized from his day of fasting. He does this on a regular basis and it is a popular method among members of his church community.

This method can even work for chronic illnesses, as Dr. Gus learned from a patient who reported curing his sarcoidosis with prayer and fasting. (Sarcoidosis is a chronic inflammatory condition, often focused in the lungs, for which conventional medicine has no cure.) Dr. Gus investigated the research and was surprised to find that pragmatic researchers have documented the emotional, spiritual and even physical benefits of prayer.

Dr. Gus describes healing prayer in the Christian tradition as praying for full restoration and healing for the patient; for guidance for the health care professionals caring for the patient; and for "understanding of what God wants us to learn from these difficult times." When counseling patients in the ICU—some of them near death, some of them having just survived a close brush with death—he suggests that they look for the "greater purpose" in their experience. Sometimes he sees these health crises bringing together family members who had become estranged, sometimes awakening people to a spiritual rebirth.

Dr. Gus describes a patient who used fasting successfully:

Natalie had seen multiple doctors and was very frustrated by the time she came to my clinic. I had a deep conversation with her about the triggers for her cough and found that it was worse when reaching out to her 20-year-old daughter, who had run away from home. Natalie began sobbing as she described how difficult it had been to raise her daughter as a single mother, compounded by her turbulent relationship with her ex-husband. She and her daughter had not spoken for months, and every time she thought of her daughter, she choked back a sob which turned into a cough.

I spoke to Natalie about the importance of forgiveness, how she and her daughter needed to forgive each other in order to heal their relationship and heal her cough. Natalie was overeating—whether to numb her feelings or fill her inner emptiness—so I talked to her about fasting and then cleaning up her diet. I suggested that she start exercising, I showed her some breathing exercises, and I taught her how to use a neti pot for her postnasal drip.

Natalie followed all these instructions, and when she came back for her three month followup, I could hardly recognize her. Her postnasal drip and her cough were gone, her daughter had moved back in, she and her daughter were going for walks together every morning, and her facial expression had totally changed to one of happiness.

The power of prayer

Larry Dossey, MD, the pioneer in studying the healing effects of prayer at a distance, has described a groundbreaking study on patients after surgery: in addition to the conventional treatments, half the patients were prayed for by people they did not even know; the results were dramatic. The prayed-for group had a lower severity score and needed less medication (antibiotics and diuretics) and less ventilatory assistance with breathing. As Dossey has observed, if a drug were discovered with these benefits, it would immediately be adopted by every hospital in America.

Yet the concept of healing prayer arouses tremendous skepticism, Dossey admits, because it challenges our view of reality. Conventional medicine has gone through three main phases in recent times, he says: the mechanical model (body as machine to be manipulated by drugs and surgery); followed in the 1970s by modern medicine's acceptance of the mind-body connection in "psychosomatic diseases"; and now "nonlocal effects," the role of consciousness, based on our interconnectedness even at a distance. We are on the cusp of this third era, as emerging evidence for nonlocal effects challenges the dominant paradigm.

This effect of prayer is clearly not based on the placebo effect, Dossey points out; most of the studies on people have been blinded (people did not know they were being prayed for), and prayer has even worked on healing animals and encouraging the growth of bacteria. In one remarkable study, half the women at a Korean fertility clinic who were having difficulty conceiving were prayed for by people in the US and Canada; they had successful pregnancies at twice the rate of the control group who were not prayed for. None of the women involved were aware of the prayer.

Dossey notes that after years of skepticism from the medical establishment, prayer is now included in the curriculum of 90 medical schools. More than a hundred research studies on prayer are summarized in Dossey's books, notably *Healing Words: The Power of Prayer and the Practice of Medicine* and *Prayer Is Good Medicine*.

Meditation

Calming the mind through meditation, we naturally feel more peaceful and tend to take more relaxed breaths. We can also develop the ability to focus our body's healing energy on a particular place or problem.

Mindfulness Meditation as taught by Dr. Jon Kabat-Zinn is well known and well-researched in hospital settings. Dr. Kabat-Zinn and his team at the UMass Medical School Center for Mindfulness deserve enormous credit for establishing the validity of meditation through research and making it an acceptable modality in mainstream medicine.

Personally, I (Burke Lennihan) have found a heart-center form of meditation to work better for me than a mind-based form. Maybe my mind is busier than most people's! As spiritual teacher Sri Chinmoy has observed, there is no one best form of meditation; however there is a kind that will work best for you, and you may need to try several different kinds to find your favorite.

If you would like to learn Mindfulness Meditation, you can readily find Dr. Kabat-Zinn's books, downloadable guided meditations and apps online. Here I will share some of my favorite heart-center meditation techniques, ones I teach at my meditation classes at Harvard University's Center for Wellness, where the challenge of calming the mind is paramount for participants.

Gently touch yourself in the middle of the breastbone, right where you point to yourself when you say, "This is me" (we don't point to our brains!). Bring your awareness to this spot and imagine your breath going in and out of this point, directly into your chest, rather than through your nose or mouth. Follow your breath as it flows into your chest, just a few inches behind where your finger is touching and a few inches in front of your spine, right in the middle of your chest. Imagine a golden glowing ball of light and love and warmth and energy. This is your heart center.

For a simple heart-centered meditation, sit with your eyes closed, listening to peaceful music if you like, and continuing to breathe slowly, deeply and gently. As you breathe in, feel that you are breathing in peace; as you breathe out, feel that you are letting go of thoughts, letting them flow out on your outgoing breath as if they are floating out on an outgoing tide.

You will get the greatest benefit from practicing this regularly, even five or ten minutes a day. You will notice yourself no longer getting upset at things (or people!) that normally irritate you or frustrate you. You will probably have fewer worries about the future and less self-criticism about the past, instead feeling more fully aware in the present and able to have positive, loving relationships with the people around you. You will see benefits within a few weeks of making meditation a daily practice.

Guided visualizations

You may be able to use a visualization to consciously overcome the cough reflex or whatever is triggering the cough. This will be easier to do in an emergency situation if you practice meditation and visualization on a daily basis. Of course you shouldn't do this if you need to cough out mucus or something else in your lungs. Sometimes, though, coughing becomes a kind of habit that you don't actually need, and this visualization can be helpful.

Let's say you feel a tickle starting to form in the back of your throat and you know that you're just about to have to cough. This is especially likely to happen when you're in the middle of a lecture or concert, which shows that it's at least partly psychosomatic! As the tickle forms, your body reacts by constricting your throat. Instead, bring your conscious awareness to that point (you're really good at this now because you've been practicing in your daily meditation) and imagine your throat relaxing and opening up. As often as the tickle/constriction comes back, visualize your throat relaxing and opening up. I've used this technique many times to overcome a cough in a situation where it would be embarrassing or distracting.

The power of meditation and guided visualization has been well documented by my friend and colleague Peggy Huddleston in her book *Prepare for Surgery, Heal Faster.* Her research at some of the most prestigious teaching hospitals in Boston shows that these techniques help people recover faster from surgery with less pain, having needed less anesthesia, and with fewer complications. In fact Huddleston is now teaching the method to cancer patients and she says it can be used for anyone suffering from any illness. While the book and accompanying guided meditation CD are essential for anyone wishing to fully master the technique, it can be summarized as

- organizing a support team of family and friends;
- learning to relax by summoning the mental image of a favorite venue where you feel deeply relaxed;
- visualizing a strongly-desired positive outcome after surgery, such as a favorite activity you will be able to resume when you recover;
- creating a positive mental attitude rather than dwelling on worries;
- repeating positive statements called affirmations (and/or having your surgical team repeat them for you while under anesthesia); and
- asking your friends and family to surround you with love and prayers while you are going through surgery. Huddleston describes this as the "pink blanket of love."

There is much more to the method, of course. Physiological reasons for the powerful effects of this deceptively simple method include the decreased blood loss when the person is relaxed. When someone is under stress, the "fight-or-flight" mechanism constricts blood vessels and increases heart rate and blood pressure. This can cause blood flow to more than double, so that more blood is lost during surgery. If the same person is relaxed during surgery, substantially less blood will be lost—explaining this benefit of the "Prepare for Surgery" method in research studies. This is just one of many physical benefits documented in the book and on the website www.healfaster.com.

Affirmations

Affirmations are statements in the present tense that set a positive intention for the future. You can create your own based on specific goals for health or you can use the famous original affirmation by Emile Coué published more than 100 years ago:

"Every day in every way I am getting better and better."

Choosing a health goal for yourself is good but it can also be limiting. Maybe you could learn a particular lesson from a health condition before you overcome it. Or maybe you could end up healthier overall as it forces you to change to a healthier lifestyle. Simply envisioning that a health condition has disappeared might not be the best for you in the big picture. Coué's affirmation allows the healing energy to go where it is needed, without your directing it or choosing a specific outcome.

Here are more suggestions for saying it effectively:

- ∾ Just let the words play through your mind.
- ∾ Do not engage your will; say it as if you don't mean it.
- ∾ Say it 20 times (or more) before falling asleep.
- ∾ You can use a string with 20 beads or 20 knots in it if you like; many people fall asleep before they get to 20.
- ∾ Say it again 20 times on waking.

You can also let it run if you have any other times when your mind isn't occupied during the day. This way those healing thoughts will settle into your unconscious.

You can find dozens of Louise Hay's inspiring affirmations on her website, www.LouiseHay.com/affirmations. You will find affirmations for health ("I am pain free and totally in sync with my life," "I love every cell of my body") as well as for spiritual inspiration ("My day begins and ends with gratitude and joy," "I am one with the very Power that has created me.")

You will find many more affirmations on her website, beautifully illustrated, and you may be inspired to create your own. Someone with breathing problems, for example, might say, "I breathe freely and easily" to help create a positive intention for better breathing. Or you could choose to repeat a statement that blends physical health with spiritual upliftment such as "I breathe in peace with each inhale; I offer gratitude with each exhale." The idea is to find a phrase or sentence that inspires you, that flows easily whether you say it aloud or silently, and then to repeat it many, many times a day.

Forest walking

Did you know that in Japan, walking in the pine woods is used as a treatment for depression? It makes intuitive sense—walking in the woods combines exercise, fresh air, and breathing in the pine fragrance, all "natural antidepressants." The Japanese have even done research on what they call *shinrinyoku* or "forest bathing" as a substitute for antidepressants.

You can also say your prayers or repeat your affirmations while walking in the woods. It's called multitasking with your mind-body methods!

Your Shortcut Guide to Mind-Body Methods

Take a few minutes for one of the practices in this chapter. Dr. Gus tells his patients that it will be the most pleasant minutes of their day. The easiest way to start might be by listening to our guided meditations on our website. The other methods are certainly worth taking the time to learn and practice. Consider them an investment in your health—an investment of your precious time.

✎ EIGHT ✎

DayQuil, NyQuil, WhatQuil?
Choosing the Appropriate
Over-the-Counter Product

It was a rainy South Florida winter day, and the temperature had dropped to a "low" 65°. Every South Floridian in the town of Weston took the opportunity to break out the leather coats. Nicole, my precious wife, was no exception. Geared up in her winter wear, she dashed off to the local pharmacy.

There, standing in the cough medicine aisle, was a biker dressed in black leather. He looked miserable. He constantly cleared his throat and swiped a finger under his nose to catch the drips. From the corner of her eye she noticed that he would pick up a box (sometimes three at a time), read the label and put it back. He did this countless times. Finally he put them all back, rolled his eyes, and let out a loud sigh of sheer frustration. My beautiful wife, always willing to help, commented, "You don't know which one to choose, huh?"

"Yeah."

"I know how frustrating that can be," she said.

"I'm frustrated all right—this is the third time I've come to the pharmacy in two weeks, with the same symptoms, and I still haven't gotten the right medication. They just don't seem to be helping."

With a compassionate smile she responded, "Don't worry. I'll help you figure it out. More importantly, I'll help you save time and money by showing you how to read the labels."

"Are you a doctor?" he asked.

"No, my husband is—and he specializes in coughs. He's written about you," she replied.

"About me?"

"Well, not literally about you, but people like you who struggle when it comes to choosing the appropriate medication. I know for a fact that oftentimes when we ask the pharmacist, they point to a group of medications on the shelf and you end up buying an ad-driven one."

"Oh, you don't know the half of it," he said. "I've visited Urgent Care twice in the past two weeks. I took the antibiotics they prescribed and the cough suppressants and I'm still the same."

"Ugh, that's terrible. Look here, let me show you, the front cover is just an eye-catching name that displays certain symptoms. Companies change the name of the medication as they wish. For example, the active components of Robitussin can be found under a different brand name from companies such as Target, Wal-Mart, CVS, Walgreens, and others. Are you bringing up phlegm?"

"No, I just have this dry persistent cough with a tickle in my throat. Otherwise, I'm fine."

"Well, my husband says antihistamines are all people need for that kind of a cough." She picked a generic antihistamine and handed it to him. "You see," she said, pointing to the shelf, "brand names are more expensive than generics and they have same active ingredients. This is what my husband recommends." He smiled and seemed grateful for the quick lesson.

Let's take a closer look and let me break down the puzzling world of over-the-counter drugs (OTCs) for you.

Solving the OTC conundrum

The over-the-counter drug market for coughs and colds is in dire need of overhaul from the Food and Drug Administration (FDA). However, even if the FDA intervenes, another problem with OTC cough-and-cold medications will still remain: the general public has not been educated in how to choose the right one.

In fact, even the experts in the field are not well informed! I recently saw a good friend, a renowned pulmonologist, give his kids Robitussin for a very mild cough. I couldn't believe it. Robitussin Children's Cough & Cold is a combination of three medications (dextromethorphan, guaifenesin, and phenylephrine) with significant side effects — and *no research proving their individual effectiveness!*

Unfortunately, *not a single medical school, residency, or fellowship training offers a course in OTCs,* and this is why even physicians may not know all the facts. But it's not rocket science. Folks at all levels of education assume that just because products are on the pharmacy shelves, they are safe and effective, but often they are not. With this book I hope to open the doors and unravel, decipher, expose, and demystify the conundrum of OTCs.

I recommend trying the natural approach first, however if that is too much of a stretch for you, this chapter will teach you the safest and most effective OTCs. Trying to choose the appropriate OTCs can be overwhelming, but when you apply my principles, it all becomes a whole lot easier (see summary table on pages 134–137 for details):

- If and when you use OTCs, choose remedies based on the predominant symptoms, avoiding combination medicines that have ingredients you do not need.
- OTCs can be taken in combination with natural remedies and/or homeopathic medicines for optimal results.
- I recommend an antihistamine (such as Claritin, Allegra, Zyrtec, or Benadryl) and a low dose of Tylenol (less than 1500 mg a day total of acetaminophen), plus a saline nasal spray if your nose is stuffed up. You can learn about other OTCs that have to be used with more caution from our table on pages 134–137.

Reading the label

Reading medication labels can be a challenge. Perhaps "a challenge" is an understatement. First of all, I know that reading the active ingredients (the part of the medications that are effective) may be like trying to read a foreign language. I guess that in order for the names to be impressive, they have to be unpronounceable and confusing. That said, let's go ahead and dive into the label.

Every drug label has two sides — front and back, let's call them part A and part B. Part A has something catchy, easy to read and to remember, and lists what the medication claims to be for: fever, itchy nose, cough, stuffy nose, runny nose, and so forth.

Pharmaceutical companies know that the average consumer can't recognize or pronounce the scientific name of the active ingredient, so they promote their own brand names: Tylenol instead of acetaminophen, Bayer instead of salicylic acid, NyQuil instead of dextromethorphan. They use catchy jingles and slogans to help you remember their product. "Plop-plop-fizz-fizz, oh what a relief it is!" If that makes you think of Alka-Seltzer, then their marketing job was well done. Or how about "The sniffling, sneezing, coughing, aching, stuffy head, fever, so-you-can-rest medicine"? NyQuil, of course. Remember, just because it's catchy and cute doesn't mean the drug works.

You probably have a busy lifestyle and want to get in and out of the pharmacy in five milliseconds, so you may be tempted to make your decision based only on part A of the label. This side is easy to read and you identify with it because it lists the symptoms it claims to work for. But if you don't read part B, you'll run into three crucial problems:

- ∾ **First,** you run the risk of **taking medications that you don't need** by choosing an ad-driven combination.
- ∾ **Second,** by not choosing a symptom-specific medication you end up going back and forth to the pharmacy for a different product in hopes it will work, but in reality it's the same medication with a different name. **Taking too much of the same active ingredient** can cause side effects and even an overdose, which can be fatal (for example in the case of Tylenol: see page 6).
- ∾ **Third,** you may end up **paying more for a brand name** because, of course, the advertising company has done its job. Next time

you're in the pharmacy, look for the generic form right next to the advertisement-driven brand. The generic is just as effective. Compare the brand name with the generic one and you will find the same "active ingredients." You will learn more about "active ingredients" as we get into part B of the label.

Part B of the label is the one with the active ingredients, side effects, cautions, and dosages. Most people turn the box over and read part B just to glance at the dosage. However, this is the area that deserves your attention.

It's very simple. Out of more than 3,000 over-the-counter products for coughs and colds, you only need to remember two groups of active ingredients: "antihistamine" and "pain reliever/fever reducer." More than 60% of all OTC medications for cough and cold are a combination of these two groups. In fact, these two groups can relieve 90% of all cough and cold symptoms. You don't even need the others. It is very important to understand that these medications should never be the first line treatment—your number one resource should be our suggested natural approach.

On the next page, I will introduce you to part B of the drug label. But first, a caution about not taking too much of a medicine. I know this not only through my medical education, but also through personal experience. This is a true story.

Meet grandpa Miguel, a little old man adopted by many in our small town as their grandfather. Grandpa was in his sixties when he went to the doctor complaining of a cough and stuffy, runny nose. The doctor assessed him and prescribed diphenhydramine tablets (Benadryl). He rushed to the pharmacy but they only had it in syrup form. (In socialist Cuba, you don't have options.)

Grandpa put his bottle of antihistamine in his pocket and went out to the street to flag down a truck, car, or horse and buggy, pretty much whatever came his way (Cuba's public transportation to this day). While waiting he took a sip, the medication went down easy, and he thought, "One tablespoon every eight hours? Hmm … maybe if I drink it all at once, I'll feel better faster." By the time he got home he had drunk the entire bottle. Shortly thereafter he was fast asleep … for the next 18 hours! His wife thought he had a stroke and rushed him to the hospital. They spent the entire night there just to find out that it was a medication overdose.

Drug Facts

(1)

Active ingredient (in each tablet)   Purpose
Chlorpheniramine maleate 2 mg . . . . .Antihistamine

(2)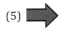

Uses temporarily relieves these symptoms due to hay fever or other upper respiratory allergies:
- sneezing   ■ runny nose   ■ itchy, watery eyes
- itchy throat

(3)

Warnings
Ask a doctor before use if you have
- glaucoma
- a breathing problem such as emphysema or chronic bronchitis
- trouble urinating due to an enlarged prostate gland

Ask a doctor or pharmacist before use if you are taking tranquilizers or sedatives.

When using this product
- you may get drowsy   ■ Avoid alcoholic drinks
- Alcohol, sedatives, and tranquilizers may increase drowsiness
- Be careful when driving a motor vehicle or operating machinery
- Excitability may occur, especially in children

If pregnant or breastfeeding, as a health professional before use.
Keep out of use of children. In case of overdose, get medical help or contact a Poison Control Center right away.

(4)

Directions

Adults and children 12 years and over	Take 2 tablets every 4 to 6 hours; not more than 12 tablets in 24 hours
Children 6 years To under 12 years	Take 1 tablets every 4 to 6 hours; not more than 6 tablets in 24 hours
Children under 6 years	Ask a doctor

(5)

Other information Store at 20-25°C (68-77°F)
- protect from excessive moisture

(6)

Inactive Ingredients D&C yellow no.10, lactose, magnesium stearate, microcrystalline cellulose, pregelatinized starch

Now that you know why you have to pay attention to warnings and dosage instructions, I will introduce you to the parts of the drug label, illustrated on the left.

1. **Active ingredient:** This hard-to-pronounce name is the actual medication. Read this name along with its purpose: this is what you're actually looking for. Drug companies put whatever name they want on the front, but if the active ingredient is the same, you can save money by buying the generic.

2. **Uses:** Highlights the symptoms *temporarily* relieved by this medication. As you can see above, an antihistamine treats most symptoms associated with acute cough and cold in the absence of pain.

3. **Warnings:** Please pay attention! Most people never read the warnings or contraindications (i.e. reasons not to use the drug). We physicians see people in the ER with painful or even dangerous complications from drug side effects, like urinary retention or glaucoma from cough suppressants or antihistamines. I have seen patients with hallucinations and insomnia from phenylephrine (a component of Robitussin) incorrectly diagnosed as having Alzheimer's.

4. **Directions:** This is the dosage (how much to take) and frequency (how often). It should be considered the *maximum* amount. Sometimes folks assume that if they take more than the recommended dosage they will feel better faster—NOT so! Not only can you feel worse, you may suffer major side effects.

    You don't have to take as much as the label says. Use common sense. If you feel better, stop taking the medication. This only applies to over-the-counter drugs, though. Don't stop your prescription medication!

5. **Other information:** This is usually reserved for the recommended temperature for storage.

6. **Inactive ingredients:** These can include sugars, alcohol, and other chemicals added to the active ingredients to create the tablet, protect it from degrading, facilitate absorption, and/or to make a lozenge or

syrup tastier. The alcohol in cough syrups used to create problems with alcohol addiction and withdrawal, less so now because very few people are using alcohol-based syrups. However, people deliberately using cough syrups as a source of alcohol can still develop all the side effects including confusion, hallucinations, and even death.

Moreover, alcohol banned from medicines in the US is widely used in other countries because it is inexpensive. I frequently see people in my clinic who have brought back alcohol-based cough syrups from other countries. Children are especially vulnerable to them.

> AVOID cough syrups that contain alcohol. They can contain as much as 20% alcohol; this is half the alcohol concentration of whiskey. Alcohol may suppress the cough reflex by inducing sedation. Most cough syrups may also contain high levels of sugar. If given in excess, they can cause diarrhea. Syrups should not be given to breastfed infants, as the sugar they contain may suppress an infant's appetite for breast milk.
>
> For more than 25 years the World Health Organization has recommended reducing alcohol in medications as much as possible.

Now let's take a look at different types of cough medications. Do they work? Are they dangerous? Here's the story.

Cough suppressants

Drugstore shelves are packed with over-the-counter cough medications promising quick relief, yet most people find themselves going back to the pharmacy again and again, searching for a brand that works. Some people report that brand X worked last year but not this year, while others get attached to a specific brand and take it throughout an acute cough/

flu episode even when they find no significant improvement. Remember that the symptoms of a viral infection can change every few days, and also viruses can mutate quickly. That's why a particular brand may work one year but not the next.

One of the nation's most distinguished experts on coughs (Dr. Richard Irwin, chairman of the Cough Guidelines Committee of the American College of Chest Physicians and editor of the journal *CHEST*) stated in an NBC News interview, "Despite the billions of dollars spent every year in this country on over-the-counter cough syrups, most such medicines do little, if anything, to relieve coughs."

Furthermore, according to Dr. Irwin, "The best studies that we have to date would suggest there's not a lot of justification for using these medications because they haven't been shown to work.... Over-the-counter cough syrups generally contain drugs in too low a dose to be effective, or contain combinations of drugs that have never been proven to treat coughs."

And how about the unintended consequences of these medications? Clinical research hasn't proven their power but our youngsters have. According to the prevention campaign StopMedicineAbuse.org, a third of all teens know someone who has abused OTC cough drugs to get high.

Robert Earl, also known as "DJ Screw," popularized a lethal cocktail called "purple drank" or "sizzurp." It consists of two readily available over-the-counter medications—codeine found in cough syrups and promethazine, an antihistamine—plus a fruit-flavored soda and a Jolly Rancher hard candy. The concoction is confirmed to have killed several prominent users, including DJ Screw himself and his understudy Big Moe. It is widely considered a source of "inspiration" for the "chopped and screwed" style of hip-hop music.

This combination can depress the brain and breathing, producing cardiorespiratory arrest (stopping the heart and lungs). Users can also experience nausea, dizziness, impaired vision, memory loss, hallucinations, and seizures. The National Institute on Drug Abuse says,

"Teens may think that just because something is available from the pharmacy, it won't harm them—but that's not true."

And cough suppressants don't even work for their intended use—the codeine-like dose is too low. Any antihistamine will work better than any cough suppressant. Let's explore the antihistamines: their pros and cons and my top recommendations.

Antihistamines

Out of all the over-the-counter medications, this is the only group I usually recommend to my patients for the treatment of acute coughs. Histamine, a chemical circulating in our blood stream, is responsible for fluid leaking out of very small blood vessels into the surrounding tissue. It gets activated when tissue in the stomach and/or the respiratory system is exposed to an allergen. The nose, the gatekeeper for the lungs, is the first responder with runny nose (fluid leaking out the blood vessels), and stuffy nose (from the tissue inflammation). The antihistamine blocks the histamine, thus decreasing the secretion and inflammation and thereby improving the cough, nasal stuffiness, watery eyes, and dripping sensation in the back of the throat.

The earliest group or "first generation" of OTC antihistamines was diphenhydramine (Benadryl) and chlorpheniramine (Chlor-Trimeton). The second generation includes loratadine (Claritin), cetirazine (Zyrtec) and fexofenadine (Allegra). Other forms of antihistamines, such as topical and intranasal, are only available by prescription.

The first generation produces stronger side effects, such as drowsiness, disturbed coordination, respiratory depression, blurred vision, urinary retention, excessive dryness, and thickening of the respiratory secretions. Long-term use can even contribute to dementia and Alzheimer's, according to recent research.

The second generation of drugs produces milder side effects but they are less effective. In order to avoid the stronger side effects of the first generation, I suggest you try the milder ones first as they may suffice. Then again, these side effects do not occur in everyone. Some people are less sensitive than others. For example, I have some patients who have been taking diphenhydramine (Benadryl) for more than 10 or even 20 years without significant side effects.

This is also the only group I sometimes recommend to my patients, out of all the over-the-counter medications, for the treatment of coughs triggered by postnasal drip. Antihistamines work by stopping the postnasal drip. However, you can accomplish the same results with our recommended herbal and homeopathic products, which work without side effects. Use the recommended antihistamine only when you have tried our natural remedies and found no relief.

"PM" medications (sleep-inducing)

Most OTCs that say "PM" on the label contain a combination of acetaminophen (Tylenol) or ibuprofen (Advil) with diphenhydramine (Benadryl). The latter is meant to make you drowsy while the others help you sleep by relieving pain. But diphenhydramine (Benadryl) is never recommended as a sleeping aid by sleep medicine doctors because of its side effects, including making sleep apnea worse. In fact many people who take "PM" combination medications as a sleeping aid are unaware of the potential harmful side effects from the other drugs in the mix, which they most likely do not even need. These medications should be completely avoided. I strongly recommend natural alternatives for sleep such as herbal teas or Calms Forte (see page 141) when necessary.

Topical anesthetic agents (for sore throats)

Topical anesthetics (benzocaine, for example in Cepacol Sore Throat, and dyclonine, for example in Sucrets Sore Throat) are used to provide temporary relief of sore throat pain by numbing the nerve endings. They are available mainly as oral lozenges, but also as aerosols, gels, or solutions. Many also include an antiseptic such as one of the phenols, alcohol, cetylpyridinium, or quaternary ammonium compounds—chemicals *intended* to kill bacteria. However, no research has proven that these chemicals are actually *effective* in fighting viral or bacterial infections.

> **Warning!** Anesthetics should not be used in young children and adults with swallowing problems because of the risk of aspiration (breathing a substance into the lungs, which can cause choking or a lung infection). Young children usually cannot gargle without ingesting the medicine. If they swallow these medications, they will experience significant side effects including nausea and irregular heartbeat. We recommend refraining from using them. There is no research study proving efficacy (whether they work in suppressing the cough), safety (side effects), the safe daily dosage, and the safety of long-term use.

Topical antitussives (agents that suppress a cough, applied to the skin)

Vicks VapoRub is the best known example. The two most popular and widely used antitussive ingredients are camphor and menthol made from plant essential oils. Menthol has been used for centuries in Asia and India for mint flavoring and for topical medical applications. Camphor is also one of the most popular OTCs with a wide range of uses, primarily as a topical remedy. People use it primarily for the treatment of coughs, but it is also used to treat itching, pain, arthritis, cold sores, and hemorrhoids. (Vicks originally used the essential oil but now uses synthetic camphor.)

During an acute cough most people apply a thin layer around the chest and neck area and/or nose and some inhale it. There isn't a specific method of use that has been studied and there is no evidence of prolonged benefit in treating coughs. In medicine, we want proof of effectiveness from scientific studies. Camphor and menthol have none of that, yet they are present in almost every home in America. That's the case in my house — my mom uses Vicks on my children every time they have a cough. She rubs it on their neck, chest, nostrils, and even on the soles of their feet! This produces local vasodilation (dilating the blood vessels), thereby increasing the blood flow. It gives a sensation of coldness that reduces pain and the urge to cough.

I have explained to my patients and family the dangers of putting this type of ointment into the nostrils. I always tell them about a patient I have with fibrosis (scar tissue) in the lungs, on the verge of a lung transplant because she frequently applied these products inside her nose. I had another patient who would apply menthol in her nose every night before going to bed for several years. She said it helped her fall asleep. Twenty years later she developed a dry cough, followed by shortness of breath on exertion. When she came to my clinic, I diagnosed scar tissue in her lungs as well — quite a severe side effect from a medication commonly considered harmless.

Nonmedicated lozenges

Nonmedicated lozenges such as Hall's or any of the store brands are very popular. They may temporarily relieve the cough by increasing production of saliva, giving the sensation of coolness and less irritation. However, no research studies have proven their value. They are probably the most widely used placebos in America. In fact, they can often cause heartburn (acid reflux) which in turn can worsen the cough. They should be avoided in young children due to the risk of aspiration (breathing them into the lungs), plus they have high sugar content. You can get the same effect with saline gargles and better results with the herbal lozenges on page 60.

Expectorants (drugs that help you cough up mucus from your lungs)
What can I say about guaifenesin? There is limited research to support
the use of guaifenesin (contained in Robitussin, Mucinex and Humibid).
I have never used it. Labels claim it loosens thick secretions. However,
there is no research study proving the efficacy or safety of this medication.
Its popularity comes from the absence of an effective pharmaceutical
competitor. Better to use an enzyme-based mucus-thinner like Mucostop,
or water and vitamin C-rich fresh juices, like lemon juice in hot water.

Oral decongestants (drugs that decrease mucus in your nose)
Ephedrine and pseudoephedrine are present in most of the OTCs
containing the "D" or "fed" suffix, such as Actifed, Sudafed, Aleve–D,
Allegra–D, Claritin–D, and Mucinex–D, as well as Benadryl Plus,
Theraflu and many others. They temporarily relieve nasal congestion and
cough associated with postnasal drip. However, their side effects are rapid
and problematic. They stimulate the central nervous system, producing
high blood pressure, anxiety, tremors, insomnia, and rapid heartbeat.
Hallucinations, seizures, and strokes have even been reported.

Pseudoephedrine is used in the illegal drug market to create
amphetamines. It is for this reason that the US and many other countries
have created strict laws prohibiting or carefully regulating its sale. I always
refrain from recommending any OTC containing the active ingredients
ephedrine or pseudoephedrine.

A similar ingredient, phenylephrine, is now being used instead, for
example in combinations like Sudafed PE. It's supposed to be safer than
the others, but it can be dangerous when combined with acetaminophen/
tylenol. This combination shows up a lot so you really have to scrutinize
the back of your medicine label! The acetaminophen quadruples the level
of phenylephrine in your blood, which greatly increases the risk of side
effects—which include rapid heart rate, difficulty breathing, dizziness,
anxiety, weakness, fever, chills, body aches and flu symptoms—probably
some of the symptoms you were taking it for in the first place!

Intranasal decongestants (mucus-thinning nasal sprays)
Oxymetazolin (Afrin), phenylephrine (Sudafed) and xylometazoline (Triaminic) are temporarily effective at relieving nasal congestion. However, when you stop using them, the congestion comes back worse than before (known as "rebound congestion"). This prompts folks to use them over and over until they develop burning and irritation of the nostril. At this point they have developed something called "rhinitis medicamentosa"—a fancy term for "nasal congestion caused by medication." Actually it can include much worse symptoms such as a chemical burn of the nostril. A large number of patients find themselves at our cough clinic due to these side effects.

Analgesics, anti-inflammatories, and **antipyretics** (fever-lowering drugs)
Analgesics (pain medications such as aspirin, acetaminophen/Tylenol and ibuprofen) are seldom recommended by themselves for acute cough or flu. However, BE AWARE that they are usually mixed in with multiple over-the-counter combination drugs for other symptoms that accompany coughs or flu: muscle pain, sore throat, chest pain from coughing, and fever. For the most part, these symptoms usually go away on their own without treatment. If the symptoms are persistent or interfere with your daily routine, consider using our natural recommendations in the next chapter, which cause little to no side effects. Most natural remedies can even be given to children under six years old without any problems.

Anti-pain medications can have serious side effects. Ibuprofen (Advil, Motrin) can produce gastritis, gastric ulcers, and even bleeding. It can even damage the kidneys. Aspirin cannot be given to children because it can cause a rare but dangerous disease called Reye's syndrome.

Acetaminophen/Tylenol is one of the most common causes of liver failure and liver transplant in industrialized countries, as we have already mentioned. Anyone with a chronic liver condition should refrain from using acetaminophen. New evidence from reviewing large-scale studies reveals additional side effects, including the disruption of thyroid and female hormonal function. In addition, when taken in pregnancy or given in infancy it can later cause asthma plus neurodevelopmental and behavioral disorders in children, including attention deficit hyperactivity disorder.

For these reasons, I recommend only taking these medications when the pain is so severe that it limits your life in some way. For example, if you are suffering from a severe sore throat and it's limiting your ability to talk, or it's so bad that you cannot sleep, then I suggest you take them. However, you can first try one of the natural pain relievers recommended in the next chapter.

If you have to use acetaminophen, use good judgment. The label may say "take every six hours" but that does not mean you have to keep taking it! Remember to only take it "as needed." If the pain has subsided after the first dose, just wait; that may be enough. Each time you are due for another dose, stop and ask yourself if your pain or fever is tolerable. If you can get by without it, skip that dose.

On the following four pages is a table summarizing the most popular OTCs with excellent pearls to refer to.

Dr. Gus's recommendations

The painful reality is that most of these medications have minimal or no scientific evidence for their use. They have too many side effects and the risk of complications outweighs the benefits. I wholeheartedly recommend the side-effect-free natural treatments provided in this book. If you are ever in need of an over-the-counter medication, please follow our recommendations.

- ∾ Refrain from combination products.
- ∾ Antihistamines are more than enough for symptom relief of cough and flu-like symptoms.
- ∾ Try the milder antihistamines first, only resorting to the stronger ones — with stronger side effects — if the mild ones do not work (see page 124).

∾ A saline rinse is harmless and can be used to clear a stuffed up nose.

Ibuprofen (Motrin, Advil) and aspirin are acceptable to reduce fever, using them short term and only as needed. Aspirin should not be used for children because of the danger of Reye's syndrome (a rare but serious condition). Ibuprofen should not be used for *anyone* on an ongoing basis as side effects are extensive: upset stomach, gastritis, gastric ulcer, and gastric bleeding. Acute kidney injury and easy bleeding can follow.

I suggest using Tylenol and only when needed — surely not around the clock and no more than 1500 mg of acetaminophen a day, for short term use. Ibuprofen can be used instead only when necessary — for pain caused by inflammation, for quick relief from a high fever — but be sure to stop either drug as soon as the symptoms stop. Do not take either drug preventively!

In the long run, try to use the natural remedies in the next chapter instead.

	Active ingredients	Brand names	Functions
Antihistamines	First generation: Diphen-hydramine, Chlor-pheniramine	Benadryl, Chlortabs, Unisom, Vicks Zzzquil	Inhibit mucus secretion in the nasal passages, leading to decongestion. Block histamine. Good for allergic rhinitis (runny nose from allergies).
	Second generation: Loratidine, Ceti-rizine, Fexofenadine	Claritin, Zyrtec and Allegra Combination products: Claritin D, Zyrtec D, Allegra D, etc	Block histamine, decrease nasal congestion.
Saline Nasal Sprays	Normal saline	Ocean Nasal Spray, Ayr Nasal, or Little Noses	Moisten irritated mucosal membranes and loosen encrusted mucus.
Expectorants	Guaifenesin 200-400 mg every 6 to 8 hours. Maximum daily dosage 2.4g	*(Single ingredient formulations: guaifenesin)* Humibid Maximum strength, Mucinex, Robitussin *(Combination products: guaifenesin/ dextromethorphan)* Mucinex DM, Robitussin DM, Cheracol D-Cough	Apparently loosen and thin lower respiratory tract secretions making minimally productive coughs more productive.

Do they work?	When do I use them?	Side effects	Nuggets
They do! But side effects are worse than second generation so do not try first.	Nasal congestion from postnasal drip and allergic rhinitis	Drowsiness, disturbed coordination, respiratory depression, blurred vision, urinary retention, dry mouth, or dry respiratory secretions	May make existing health conditions worse (narrow angle glaucoma, peptic ulcers, bladder neck obstruction, and asthma).
NOT as much as the first generation do but side effects are milder, so try first.	Mild postnasal drip, stuffiness and nasal dripping	Similar to first generation but milder and less frequent	Not a good choice for the management of moderate cough associated with postnasal drip and nasal obstruction
Unclear efficacy but makes you feel good!	Nasal congestion, sinusitis, dry winter sinuses in adults and children	Slight burning or stinging sensation upon instillation	May be used as adjunct to specific treatment
No proven efficacy	Not recommended. This may cause you more coughing. Use *Cough Cures* recommendations instead.	Generally well tolerated; however, nausea, vomiting, dizziness, headache, rash, diarrhea, and stomach pain have been noted.	Not for chronic cough associated with lower respiratory tract diseases, asthma, COPD, emphysema, or smoker's cough.

	Active ingredients	Brand names	Functions
Oral Decongestants	Phenylephrine	Sudafed PE	Blood vessel constriction that opens the nasal passages
	Ephedrine	Primatene	Blood vessel constriction that opens the nasal passages
	Pseudo-ephedrine	*Single product:* Sudafed. *Combination products:* Claritin D, Zyrtec D, Allegra D, etc.	Blood vessel constriction that opens the nasal passages
Intranasal Decongestants	Oxy-metazoline, xylo-metazoline	Afrin, 4-way, Neo-Synephrine, and Vicks Sinex	Sudden blood vessel constriction that opens the nasal passages

Do they work?	When do I use them?	Side effects	Nuggets
Questionable efficacy	*Temporary* relief of nasal and eustachian tube congestion and cough associated with postnasal drip.	Increased **blood pressure,** stimulation of the central nervous system (anxiety, insomnia, tremors, restlessness or hallucination), and cardiovascular stimulation	Least effective of all oral decongestants. Repeated dosing may result in decreased efficacy.*
Effective but too many side effects	*Temporary* relief of nasal congestion	Increased **blood pressure,** stimulation of the central nervous system (anxiety, insomnia, tremors, restlessness or hallucination), and cardiovascular stimulation	Slowest onset and longest duration of action. Repeated dosing may result in decreased efficacy.*
Effective but too many side effects	*Temporary* relief of nasal congestion	Increased **blood pressure,** stimulation of the central nervous system (anxiety, insomnia, tremors, restlessness or hallucination), and cardiovascular stimulation	Not a good choice for the management of moderate cough associated with postnasal drip and nasal obstruction.*
Effective but at a very high price (bad side effects)	*Temporary* relief of nasal congestion	Slight burning or stinging sensation upon instillation. Produces a worsening of the inflammation, a condition called **rhinitis medicamentosa.**	Labeled as safe if stopping after 4-5 days but in reality no one is able to. Creates dependency.

*Sale restricted by the Combat Methamphetamine Epidemic Act: purchase behind the counter.

NINE

Fever, Pain and Sleep:
Now What Do I Do?

We have to treat medications like Tylenol with respect. Because they are so powerful, we need to use them sparingly. A lot of people take them like candy! Save them for when you really need them, by trying something natural first.

Let's start with fever: do we even need to treat a fever? It's an important part of the body's immune system. Physicians are currently questioning whether it's wise to treat a fever or "let it ride," even for patients who are critically ill.

How high can a fever go before it's possibly dangerous? We've asked our colleagues at the American Academy of Pediatrics to share their fever guidelines, on the next page. But first, some wise words from Miranda Castro, CCH, one of the world's most respected homeopathy authors.

Fevers in Children *by Miranda Castro, CCH*
Caring for a sick child can be a frightening experience for a parent, especially if a fever is involved. Don't panic! Fevers are not all bad. In fact, medical research over the past twenty years has consistently shown them to actually help in fighting infections.

A *weak* child may be endlessly "sick," neither very ill nor very well, but with no significant rise in temperature. A more *robust* child whose temperature soars may look and feel very ill, therefore giving more cause for concern, but is usually ill for a shorter time and recovers more quickly.

A high temperature generally indicates that the body's defense mechanism is fighting an infection and temperature variations indicate how it is coping. During a fever many of the body's natural healing processes and all the metabolic functions are speeded up. The heart beats faster, carrying the blood more quickly to all the organs; breathing is quickened, increasing oxygen intake; and sweating increases, helping the body to cool down naturally.

Often the first symptom that your child is ill is a fever. Fevers can be a helpful and necessary healing stage of an acute illness ... something positive, to be encouraged rather than suppressed. Attempts to control a fever with fever-reducing medications are likely to confuse the body's natural efforts to heal itself and can prolong an infection. Many doctors are now suggesting that a moderate fever be left to "run its course."

The basics: The average normal temperature in a healthy human is said to be 98.6°F (37°C), but this can vary. Most people, adults and children, can run a fever of up to 104°F (40°C) for several days with no danger. It is normal for healthy children to throw high fevers 103°F (39.5°C) and higher with an infection.

Take the temperature with a thermometer, tucked under the armpit for 5 minutes, for an accurate reading. It will read about a half degree Fahrenheit lower than that taken under the tongue. A fever strip (for the forehead) is a rough guide only and a hand held on the forehead is next to useless; babies that feel hot to the touch can have a normal temperature. The newer digital thermometers are much easier for young children and give a quick and accurate reading. (Always keep a spare battery in the house!)

Fevers usually peak towards night-time and drop by the following morning, so that if your child has a temperature of 104°F (40°C) in the evening it may recur on subsequent evenings. A drop in temperature in the morning does not mean that the fever is past its peak. Don't worry if it rises and falls several times over several days before finally returning to normal.

Following are the guidelines for treating fever from the American Academy of Pediatrics (AAP). Miranda Castro's guidelines have been simplified to conform to the AAP guidelines.

American Academy of Pediatrics Guidelines for Fever

Call your child's doctor right away if your child has a fever and

- looks very ill, is unusually drowsy, or is very fussy
- has been in a very hot place, such as an overheated car
- has other symptoms, such as a stiff neck, severe headache, severe sore throat, severe ear pain, an unexplained rash, or repeated vomiting or diarrhea
- has immune system problems, such as sickle cell disease or cancer, or is taking steroids
- has had a seizure
- is younger than four months and has a rectal temperature of 100.4°F (38.0°C) or higher
- has a fever rising above 104°F (40°C) repeatedly for a child of any age.
- if the fever lasts more than 1 day in a child less than 2 years old
- if the fever lasts more than 3 days in a child age 2 or older.

Be prepared! In Europe, where I (Miranda Castro) come from, most working adults are allocated a certain amount of annual sick leave (for themselves, and increasingly for their children). In the US the pace is faster; there is no time to have an accident or get sick. The God of Productivity is breathing down everyone's neck most of the time. This puts a terrible pressure on parents and their children.

If you are the parent and especially if you are a working parent, you will need to prepare yourselves for the fact that your children will fall ill from time to time, especially after they start nursery or school, and will need looking after, either by you or another caregiver. It is worthwhile to plan strategies for coping with an ill child. If you aren't prepared it is easy to feel harassed and resentful when they do fall ill. The more children you have, the more prepared you will need to be as they can fall ill one after the other instead of conveniently all at once!

Look after yourself: Looking after a sick child is draining, especially if your child is very ill and/or demanding. Cancel everything that you can: your child's health comes first. Sleep when your child sleeps, don't use her nap time to catch up on the ironing. Now is not the time to worry about whether your house is neat and tidy. Ditch the housework and spend your time off doing something enjoyable or restful or both! Make sure your own cup has something in it so that you can give to your child and still have some left over for yourself.

If you neglect your own needs at this time it is easier to fall ill once your child is better. Engage the help of neighbors, friends or family to look after your child so that you can rest or get out to recharge your batteries. Make sure you eat well and get some exercise even if it is running up and down the stairs!

Negotiate with your partner so that both of you get some time off, take it in turns to do night duty or split the night into two so that you can both get a good chunk of sleep. If you are a single parent then ask a friend in so you can take a break, even if it is for half an hour to get out for a walk.

Special treatment: Sick children deserve special treatment: reassurance if they are frightened; comforting if they are in pain; distracting from an itchy rash; sponging down if they are too hot; a time of nurturing and special healing rituals. Many parents love this time when their children are willing and eager to "lean into them."

Keep excitement levels down and encourage quiet activities such as reading, drawing, playing board games, watching a little television (too much is over-stimulating) and listening to music and stories. Don't over-stimulate sick children by taking them out or by having a lot of visitors.

Be creative about nursing your sick child and about helping them with their pain. Make sure your child goes to bed early, with daytime naps if needed. Tuck your child up in bed with you if this is OK with you, as many small children will only sleep if their parent's body is near when they feel sick.

Keep notes, a health file or notebook in which you jot down the dates of your child's illnesses and any treatment as well as the effects. List possible stresses also. This will help you to map your child's patterns of illness and help you to take a more active part in their health care. Remind yourself that illness is part of life's rich tapestry and reassure your child at every stage, however little she is, that this too will pass.

Small children with fevers: Small children who develop a fever, especially infants under six months old, must be watched carefully because they are vulnerable to becoming quickly dehydrated. Encourage your child to drink plenty of fluids, preferably water, herb teas or diluted fruit juice (not sugar-sweetened juice drinks or sodas, as sugar is a stimulant), either warm or cold as desired. Don't give acidic drinks (orange or lemon juice) to a child with mumps as they will hurt sore salivary glands. Children who are reluctant to drink will often suck on a (clean!) wet sponge or flannel, especially if the water is warm, or try an ice cube or frozen fruit juice. If you are breastfeeding a sick baby continue to nurse as often as your baby asks. The breast is especially comforting at a time like this.

Finally, remember that not all fevers are from infection ... small babies can throw a low fever if they become overheated (either in hot weather or an over-heated house) and will quickly revert to normal with undressing and/or a tepid sponging down.

Homeopathy and fevers: A fever is often the first symptom of a cold, a flu, a sore throat, an earache, a childhood illness or even an episode of teething. Each baby has their own pattern of falling ill and will experience different fever symptoms. One baby will feel hot with a high fever, will kick off the covers; another will be irritable, intolerant of any disturbance and need to be kept warm; one baby will sweat profusely, be thirsty and slightly delirious; another will be dry and hot and refuse liquids. Each of these babies will need a different homeopathic remedy to help them depending on their emotional state and general symptoms. Use all the symptoms to help your baby fight their infection safely and effectively.

The remedies: It's as easy as ABC and P! (in other words, the remedies listed below). They are the first ones to think of if your baby is feverish.

Aconite For fevers coming on suddenly, often after a chill (especially from a cold wind). Your child is fine on going to bed and then wakes around midnight with a high fever. She is hot and sweaty and thirsty, kicks the covers off and then feels cold. Her cheeks alternate between being hot and red and pale and ghostly, or one cheek may be hot and red if it is a teething fever. She can also be very restless and distressed, and you suspect that she may have a pain somewhere.

Belladonna For fevers coming on suddenly. Your baby gets so hot she radiates heat. It is a dry heat (without sweating) and can alternate with chills. She may become delirious, her pupils are more dilated than usual and she may grind her teeth (if she has any!).

Chamomilla For fevers in teething babies, or those that accompany an earache or sore throat. You will recognize this one easily because your child is very hard to please, she wants to be carried constantly but even that doesn't help much. She cries and shouts a lot and may even hit. There are red, round patches on one or both cheeks. The face can be hot whilst the body is cold.

Phosphorus For fevers in babies who do not appear as ill as you would expect! Their appetite doesn't change; they play happily in spite of a moderate to high fever. They have a dry, burning fever with a thirst, especially for cold drinks.

Pulsatilla .For fevers in teething babies or those who are coming down with an infection. These babies get easily overheated, kick the covers off and then get cold. They refuse drinks and are much better for fresh air. They want to be cuddled constantly and feel better for it.

Dosage guidelines

Match one of the pictures above with your child's symptoms. You may need to consult a first aid book like mine, *The Complete Homeopathy Handbook* by Miranda Castro, if these descriptions don't match your child's collection of symptoms. Having selected a remedy:

- Give according to the urgency of the complaint i.e. every 15-30 minutes if in severe pain, less often (every 1-2 hours) if in less pain.
- Stop on improvement (this is important: a homeopathic medicine works as a trigger, stimulating the body to heal itself).
- Repeat the same remedy if the same symptoms return.
- Change the remedy if you have given about six doses and had no reaction or if the symptoms change.

A well-selected homeopathic remedy will give speedy relief, without side effects. You might want to purchase these remedies to have on hand for those middle-of-the-night times when the stores are shut. First-aid homeopathic kits are an economical and convenient way to have commonly needed remedies always handy.

Dos & Don'ts!

Do

- Talk reassuringly to your baby about what is happening. The sound of your voice is comforting to them—and to you! Explain clearly (even to a baby) what is wrong and say how long the illness is likely to go on for.
- Be patient! Children who are sick can become more demanding and regress temporarily, sucking things, wetting the bed, and so on—sometimes even before the symptoms of the illness (rashes,

swollen glands etc.) appear. This will pass once they are on the road to recovery.

꙰ Keep your sick baby close to you—many babies want to be carried constantly and sleep better if they are tucked up in bed with their mothers during this time! Remind yourself that it won't last and you can re-establish a routine once she is well again.

꙰ Provide a calm environment for your feverish child. This is not a time to take her out shopping!

꙰ Encourage your baby to drink plenty of fluids, preferably water, herb teas, or diluted natural juices, or at least sips of water at frequent intervals. Older babies who are reluctant to drink will often suck on a (clean!) wet sponge or flannel, especially if the water is warm, or try an ice cube or frozen fruit juice. If you are breastfeeding a sick baby continue to nurse as often as your baby asks, as this is probably all that will be wanted. The breast is especially comforting when they are unwell.

꙰ Sponge your child down with tepid water if the fever goes above 103°F/104°F (40°C) and your child feels hot and sweaty. Expose and sponge one limb at a time until it feels cool to the touch. Dry it and replace it under the covers before going on to the next limb. This will help the temperature to drop by 1-2°F (up to 1°C) and can be repeated as often as necessary. Sponging the face and forehead alone can also give relief. Or you can immerse a feverish but not desperately ill child in a bath of tepid (not cold) water from time to time to bring down a fever. In any case keep a hot, feverish baby cool, and a chilly feverish baby (one who feels cold to the touch and shivers) warm.

꙰ Use homeopathic remedies when the fever is one of a number of symptoms, for example, when someone is clearly suffering from, say, earache, teething or a sore throat and a fever. If the first symptom to arise is a fever then wait for a while for other symptoms to surface before choosing a remedy based on all the symptoms. Contain the fever if necessary, by sponging down (see above).

꙰ Watch for signs of dehydration in infants under six months old, and especially in children who are refusing to drink or who are drinking less than usual.

Don't

- Encourage sick children to eat, especially if they don't want to. Fasting encourages the body in its process of healing. Give babies who are hungry small, light, nutritious meals such as fruit or vegetable purees, soups and oatmeal.
- Give any form of aspirin to a feverish child. This has been known to lead to dangerous, although rare, complications, in particular Reye's syndrome, which affects the brain and liver. You can use Children's Tylenol in an emergency, or if your baby seems to be in pain and you don't have a homeopathic remedy handy, but never exceed the recommended dose.

Seek help from your health care professional if

- Your child of any age has a febrile seizure. Take your child to a pediatrician or emergency room immediately. Chances are it's nothing, but there's an outside chance your child needs to see a doctor.
- There is a history of convulsions accompanying fevers in your family. Keep a close eye when your baby has a fever … it is the rapid rise in temperature that can cause a fit.
- The baby or older child is also refusing to drink, as dehydration can occur. Signs of dehydration include limpness, poor muscle tone, sunken eyes, and a sunken fontanelle (the soft spot at the top of the head where the bones of the skull come together). Small children who develop a fever, especially infants under six months old, must be watched carefully because they are vulnerable to becoming quickly dehydrated.
- There is a general lack of reaction (listlessness and limpness) and your baby is distressed, which can mean that a more serious illness (such as pneumonia or meningitis) is developing.
- You are worried and need reassurance about your sick baby—

contact your health care professional immediately, as it is always better to be on the safe side when it comes to your baby's health.

Thank you, Miranda, for that wealth of information! Here are more suggestions from coauthor Burke Lennihan.

For those of you who would like to try another natural route, essential oils can lower a fever. Peppermint and lavender are favorites. They can be diluted in a carrier oil like almond oil and massaged in to your child's skin. Peppermint tea works too. In fact you can combine the fever-lowering power of peppermint with the delights of a cool popsicle by making peppermint tea popsicles for your sick child. (You'll have to experiment to make them taste good to your kids—maybe sweetened with a little honey, agave or stevia, maybe mixed with coconut milk or yogurt.)

Natural Remedies for Pain

Did you know that aspirin is based on a Native American herb, white willow bark? The early settlers learned from the Native Americans to strip the bark from young willow trees in the spring and boil it as a tea for pain, fevers and inflammation. White willow bark comes with not only the same benefits as aspirin, but also the same cautions: don't use if you're allergic to aspirin, and don't give it to a child with fever.

Here are some other popular herbs for pain:

Boswellia is a fragrant herb from India, related to frankincense and myrrh. Like many herbs and supplements whose active ingredients are fat-soluble rather than water-soluble, it absorbs best when taken with a meal with some (healthy) fat or oil. It may take time to take effect, up to eight weeks, so it's not an on-the-spot pain reliever, but in the long run these natural pain relievers will protect your joints.

Curcumin is another herb from India; it's one of the active ingredients in turmeric, which gives curry its golden-yellow color. A recent study showed that curcumin worked as well or better than ibuprofen for arthritic knee pain, with greater patient satisfaction and fewer side effects. Finding an effective substitute for ibuprofen is important, since a recent study indicated that long-term use of ibuprofen may be in some ways as harmful to the heart as the now-banned Vioxx.

To get medicinal-strength curcumin, though, it's best not to rely on that bottle of turmeric powder that's been in your spice cabinet for years. Medicinal ingredients need to be carefully extracted and then protected from oxygen and other factors that could make them lose potency.

The best curcumin I know is made by Terry's Naturally. They use a special extraction process, then combine curcumin with boswellia and two other ingredients to give you the best of all worlds. If you want to use herbs for your pain instead of OTC medications, I would start with Curamin by Terry's Naturally. It can work pretty quickly; users report relief the same day or within a few days, and it can also provide long-term relief from joint pain.

What about homeopathic remedies for joint pain? The simplest approach is a combination of remedies made into a salve. There are several excellent products, each with its own fans. If the first one you try doesn't work for you, don't give up; try another.

Traumeel (recently re-labeled T-Relief) is the most widely used; **Topricin** is another big favorite; Castro's **Healing Cream for Joints and Muscles** is made by our contributing homeopathy expert and has my own favorite combination of remedies for stiff joints and for healing sore muscles and torn ligaments.

If you'd like to try a specific homeopathic remedy rather than a blend, here are the top remedies for joint pain.

Does it hurt to move? Do you wince if you have to take a step? Do you hold your chest still when you laugh, sneeze or cough because it hurts so much? **Bryonia** will work best for joint pain that's worse with even the slightest motion or even a little jolt, like when you take a step and put your foot down. Here are some other hints Bryonia might be your best bet: Your mouth feels dry and you're really thirsty, no matter how much you drink, and you're more grouchy than usual, wanting everyone to leave you alone. For an objective grouchiness assessment, ask your spouse!

But what if you *want* to move that stiff and painful joint? **Rhus tox.** is called the "rusty gate" remedy because people who need it try to swing their joint or limber it up until it moves easily — typically when they first get out of bed in the morning, but it could be any time they've been sitting still for awhile. It's also especially likely to help when your joint pain gets worse when the weather is damp. Rhus tox. can help whether your joint pain comes from a sprain or strain, or from arthritis (in which case it's likely to relieve the pain and stiffness but don't expect a permanent cure).

If Rhus tox. doesn't work, try its backup remedy: **Ruta grav.** Ruta shares with Rhus tox. the qualities of wanting to limber up the stiff joint and damp weather making the pain worse. Ruta really likes knees: think of them as dancing partners. If you have knee pain, Ruta is an especially good bet. If your knee goes out from under you painlessly, like when you're walking downstairs, try Ruta. It's healing for any connective tissue problem: any tendon or ligament injury, sprains and strains, plantar fasciitis, baker's cysts that form in the back of the knees, even eyestrain from too much computer use. (Those teeny weeny eye muscles have teeny weeny ligaments!)

Maybe it's not joint pain you're concerned with, but headache pain. We'll skip over the individual homeopathic remedies here, because there are so many good possible remedies it's hard to choose without help from a professional homeopath. That also means that a combination product for headaches can be hit or miss. If *your* best-matching remedy is in the formula, it may work like a charm; if it's not, you will get only minor relief at best. Fortunately these products are inexpensive. Try **Swanson's Headache Relief, Hyland's Headache** formula ("for stress and sick or nervous headaches") or **Hyland's Migraine Headache** relief.

There are great herbal and aromatherapy options for headache pain. Here's my favorite: **Migrastick** by Health from the Sun, an aromatherapy blend of essential oils applied to the forehead with a roller stick. Aromatherapy is based on the idea that fragrances can heal actual medical conditions. Sounds woo-woo, doesn't it?

But aromatherapy is well-researched and it makes sense scientifically: the scent receptors in your nose are nerve cells hard-wired into your brain with a single long nerve fiber that connects incoming information (like the scent of your fragrant essential oil) to a deep and primitive part of your brain. Aromatherapy has been used for millennia. I like it for headaches because it can work so fast, faster than the well-researched herbal remedies like **butterbur** and **feverfew** (which have slow and steady action for more permanent migraine relief).

Natural Remedies for Sleep

As for having a good night's sleep without drugs, a favorite among my clients is **Calms Forte,** a blend of homeopathic remedies including preparations of valerian and passionflower, traditional herbal remedies for sleep. You can also use these herbs as herbal tea, for example in **Nighty Night Tea**; however a few of my clients have reported a drugged feeling the next morning from valerian — like an herbal hangover! Calms Forte would not have that effect because the herbs are so dilute. Traditional Medicinals also makes a version of its Nighty Night Tea without valerian, which is milder in taste although less potent.

Gaia Herbs puts their excellent organic herbs into a **Sleep & Relax** formula as an herb tea, capsules, and a syrup for kids. It helps calm you so you can get to sleep in the first place, while their **Sleep Thru** formula is more geared to helping you sleep through the night.

Some safe, non-habit-forming homeopathic medicines for sleep

Cocculus is for jet lag and shift workers, when you need to reset your body clock. Try taking a dose before take-off and on landing, or before and after work, and again as needed whenever you feel sleepy when you're meant to be up or vice versa.

Coffea is for "tired and wired" kids, for anyone who can't get to sleep because they're so excited about what will happen the next day (Christmas, or getting married, or a big vacation), and anyone else lying in bed amped up (as if too much caffeine) with thoughts whirling around in their head.

Ignatia is called "the rehearsal remedy": it's for people who are upset about an emotional situation, who lie awake ruminating over a relationship issue, thinking of what they wish they had said or planning what they might do to that rat the next time they see him.

Nux vomica is for people who can't sleep because they have acid reflux or other indigestion issues and/or who lie awake thinking of their business deals. The stereotype of the Nux vomica person is someone

Your Shortcut Gu
for Fever

For fever
- Keep hydrated, try fruit
- Bring temperature with
- Use peppermint or laver
  massage (diluted in a m

For pain
- Boswellia and/or curcur
- T-Relief (Traumeel), Tolformation
  for Joints and Muscles a
- Headache pain: Swanso
  Headache formula or H _nd in my (Dr. Gus's) home-_
- Or a Migrastick aromat _n hills of Cuba. When I was_

For sleep _TV in town—a big black-_
- Calms Forte homeopat _as wrapped in so much tin_
- Nighty Night Tea by Ti _ve didn't get reception from_
- Gaia's Sleep & Relax or _ieighbors would come and_
- Remove electronics fro _the soap opera. Blackouts_
  before bed, use blue-lig _of the program ... pfft, no_

otion, though. Typically we
e show, some with runny
ould hear my mom talking
ht that made people sick,
andma and all the neigh-
lma carried an umbrella
n when it was not raining
nalady-maker.

e Spanish-speaking world
ight dew"). I even found
ipain in 1807: it says that

the "humidity in the air in the hours after sunset ... must be avoided, because it causes many diseases." This dreaded phenomenon — believed to be caused by the influence of the moon, the damp night air, and the drop in temperature after sunset — is blamed for coughs, flu, pneumonia and even death. To this day, Hispanics from Madrid to Latin America to the Philippines live in fear of the *sereno*.

Edna, a nurse I met while doing a fellowship at George Washington University, told me that she coughed from the cold air whenever she opened the door to her refrigerator. Many folks tend to believe that cold air and wind are responsible for carrying the viruses that somehow get us infected. This perception has been around since the beginning of time.

In Traditional Chinese Medicine, "wind" *(feng)* has been blamed for coughs and respiratory problems for thousands of years. *Fengsu Tongyi*, a Chinese almanac from 200 A.D., describes wind and changes in temperature as causes and triggers of respiratory diseases. Even to this day, many practitioners of Traditional Chinese Medicine consider "wind" as causing a disharmony that brings illness. Almost every civilization has blamed the cold and wind as the disease carrier or the trigger. Whether it's called *sereno*, "refrigerator air," or *feng*, it's the same phenomenon. But there's a difference between wind carrying the germs to you, versus cold and wind making you susceptible to germs you pick up by contact.

Myth: Exposure to cold air, wind or *sereno* caused my cough.

Facts: Most acute coughs are due to viral respiratory infections. You can catch a cold or flu by close contact with an infected person — a kiss, a hug, a cough or a sneeze — or by touching something like a doorknob, pen, or TV remote that the sick person handled. Once the virus is on your hands, it can gain entrance to your body if you touch your eyes, nose or mouth. Again, being exposed does not mean that you will get sick. It all depends on your body's ability to fight it off.

It's true that some people cough when exposed to cold air, especially during exercise, as my fellow runners tell me. They are trying to breathe deeply because they are running, but the cold air makes their air passages constrict, so they cough. This is not the same as getting sick from cold air, though.

Again, you may have noticed that in our discussion of homeopathic medicines for cough, some of them are specifically indicated for people who get sick after a cold wind or being outside in the cold air. Homeopathy historically has relied non-judgmentally on patients' report of their symptoms. We know that when people report getting sick from cold air, certain homeopathic medicines are likely to work well for them.

Myth: People get sick in winter because of the cold weather.

Fact: The cold weather is not directly responsible. Studies show that people get sick more often during the winter because they are stuck indoors in close contact with others, for example at shopping malls. Also the cold temperature increases the nasal discharge that spreads germs around, and people may be spreading germs even if they don't have any symptoms. The great majority of people who are exposed to a virus will fight it off, but they are still carriers. If they wipe their nose with their bare hands and then open a door, press an elevator button, hold onto a railing, or touch a checkout screen, they can leave the virus for others to enjoy.

Myth: I need to sweat out a fever.

Fact: You don't need to cover yourself with multiple blankets to "sweat the fever." The body tends to break out in a sweat when the fever breaks and the person is starting to get better, but forcing a sweat by making yourself really hot doesn't get you better any faster.

And in fact, you *want* a fever if you are sick! Fever is one of the body's main protective systems. When we are exposed to a massive load of viruses or bacteria, the body's defense cells are called to battle. Some release chemicals to destroy the invaders, and these chemicals are carried by the blood to the control tower (the brain), which tells the body to turn up the thermostat. The result is a high temperature, a fever, which destroys microbes and stimulates the body's defense cells to "swallow" the microbes. It increases the heart rate to mobilize your defense cells faster and it even increases your body's own natural interferon to kill viruses.

Hippocrates, the father of Western medicine, is credited with saying, "Give me the power to create a fever and I can cure all diseases."

Myth: Any fever over 99° needs to be medicated.

Facts: Normal temperature varies from 97° to 99°. Children over three and most adults can run a fever of 104°F (40°C) for three to five days without problems. However it becomes a concern when:

- Any time it is over 103°F
- When any fever lasts more than three days
- When a child under three has a fever greater than 102°F (39°C) lasting all day and night, because they can develop febrile seizures.

However, before medicating, try a natural approach: a lukewarm bath or lukewarm sponge bath and the natural methods recommended in the previous chapter. Make sure to have the person keep drinking water, as fevers can cause dehydration via sweating without the person realizing it. Defense-boosting shakes and green smoothies will provide good nutrition while being easy to digest; but if the person isn't hungry, don't force them to eat. Check the temperature regularly; it's natural for fevers to go up at night.

If the natural approach isn't working and the fever is rapidly rising into the danger zone, use acetaminophen (tylenol) sparingly. Definitely do not give children any drug containing aspirin (acetylsalicylic acid), as they can develop a dangerous disease called Reye's syndrome.

Myth: I have to get rid of all this mucus!

Facts: A cough with sticky phlegm is always troublesome, and it's true that the mucus triggers your cough. But the mucus isn't the problem, it's part of the solution. The body in its genius calls on all its defenses when viruses and bacteria invade your nose, throat and windpipe lining. The respiratory system, from the tip of your nose all the way to smallest airway in your lungs, is exposed to the outside air. In fact the lungs are the only internal organs in direct contact with the environment with all its microbes. The cell soldiers of the immune system use tissue swelling and mucus to block these invaders, to prevent them from getting into the secret temple (our bodies).

Once the immune system has the attackers under control, the inflamed tissue and mucus production are no longer needed and they disappear on their own. Americans spend millions of dollars on medications such as Mucinex to try to get rid of the phlegm, but research has proven that they don't work. Remember, as long as your body is creating mucus, it means the mucus is still needed for protection.

Your body wants to keep the mucus moving up and out, to get microbes out. If the mucus is too thick and sticky to budge, keep hydrating yourself and try NAC (page 63), the enzymes in Mucostop (page 63) or a homeopathic medicine like Kali bichromicum (page 81). They will support your healing energy and help move the mucus out with no side effects.

Myth: I need antibiotics — and if my doctor won't prescribe them, I'll go to another doctor who will.

Facts: Most coughs are caused by colds and flu, which in turn are caused by viruses, and antibiotics are powerless against viruses.

So taking one will not help you get over a cold or the flu faster. Instead, every time you take antibiotics more bacteria in your body may become resistant to the antibiotics themselves.

Research has found that when doctors over-prescribe antibiotics, resistance goes up, putting their patients at risk for antibiotic-resistant infections and also increasing the chances of spreading drug-resistant bacteria in their community. Doctors often prescribe antibiotics just because their patients demand it. I see this all the time; a lot of patients call the urgent care centers "Z-Pak clinics" after the antibiotic Zithromax. They go in with a cough and if the doctors don't prescribe it, they go clinic shopping until they find it.

But they are only hurting themselves, their immune system, and the health of their whole community. People need to stop asking their doctors for antibiotics! Offer your doctor a copy of this book instead to share all the evidence-based natural alternatives to antibiotics.

The only time antibiotics should be used is in the case of a secondary bacterial infection. (See the chart on page 23 about how you can tell when you might have this and need to go to your doctor to get checked.) Otherwise, typical colds and flu usually go away on their own and should not be treated with antibiotics.

Myth: I got sick on the plane from the recirculated air.

Facts: It is only logical to assume that a closed aircraft cabin would recycle all our viruses and bacteria when we breathe out, but research has disproved this. As my good friend, infectious disease expert Dr. Bob Freedman, puts it, "Viruses and bacteria don't have wings!"

The problem with the airplanes is the close contact with an infected person. Just imagine, I'm infected with the virus and my only symptom is a runny nose. I board a plane and immediately the dry air triggers more of a runny nose. I'm walking down the aisle with my carry-on in one hand and with the other wiping the watery drip. The next second, I find myself holding on to a seat to catch my balance. You are right behind me, in that small aisle that seems narrower each time you fly. You put your hand where I had put mine, then unconsciously you touch your face, and "bingo!" The virus found the official transport system. That's the way we get infected!

Myth: I've been coughing for two weeks. I must have bronchitis! I need antibiotics!

Facts: Coughs from flu or cold can last up to three weeks in healthy adults and children. That's right! 21 days. Usually the cough is the last symptom to go away. Most people with a persistent cough after a cold or flu have postnasal drip as a result of the damage produced by the virus to the mucosa (the membrane lining your nose and throat). This cough DOES NOT require antibiotics. In fact treating this kind of cough with antibiotics is the most common mistake made in treating an acute cough!

If your cough lasts longer than three weeks and you don't have other symptoms plus you are gradually getting better, you do not need to see your doctor and your cough does not need medication. It will most likely go away on its own. If it lasts more than four to six weeks, though, best to see your doctor.

Not only that, even if you do cough for more than three weeks and get bronchitis, most acute bronchitis is viral anyway and antibiotics will not help. Plus you probably don't even have bronchitis. It is over-diagnosed by busy doctors who don't have time to listen to your lungs properly. X-rays are not precise enough to diagnose bronchitis. Your doctor has to hear wheezing, but postnasal drip also causes wheezing, and it's hard to tell the difference.

So if you have a lingering cough, try the herbal remedies on page 68 instead.

Myth: My doctor says bed rest is best when I'm sick, so I have to stay in bed for three weeks!

Facts: Actually, exercise is best, both to prevent a cold or flu and to help you recover. You only need to rest for a day or two if you have a fever with general weakness, muscle aches and so forth. In fact, when we have patients in the Intensive Care Unit with severe respiratory failure, connected to a breathing machine through a tube in their throat, we let them rest for a day or two. But then we have them start exercising because we have found it speeds recovery with fewer complications. That's right! They exercise in bed with all the tubes! So don't let the cold or flu get you down—as soon as you feel slightly better, gear up and head out for your cardio. It's the best thing you can do.

Regular exercise keeps your immune system soldiers well trained and helps prevent flu and colds. In fact, research shows that it can cut in half the risk of getting colds and flu during the winter season. Years ago I learned from my friend and coach J. Balart that running or biking as soon as I feel cold symptoms coming on will cut the progression of the condition to its minimum. Ever since he told me that, as soon as I feel something coming on, I'll go for a run.

Myth: Over-the-counter medications for cough and stuffy nose must be OK for children, because the FDA has checked them out.

Facts: The American Academy of Pediatrics says OTCs for stuffy, runny noses, and coughs are *not* effective for kids younger than six. They even go as far to say that they can have harmful side effects. The World Health Organization (WHO) agrees that there are no effective cough and cold medications for young children, and that the OTCs have potentially harmful side effects. WHO recommends honey and lemon, tamarind tea, and other simple home remedies like those in this book.

Myth: I should go the doctor as soon as I have cold symptoms … just in case.

Facts: Coughs and cold are one of the most common reasons for doctor's office visit, but the great majority of these visits are preventable. The doctor will only prescribe antibiotics, which are both ineffective and potentially harmful. The only reasons you need to call the doctor are those covered in the safety guidelines on page 23.

Myth: Kids in daycare catch more colds than other children.

Facts: The endless fountain of mucus running down the nose and making its way to the mouth and chin is the daily picture of a child in daycare—known as the "daycare syndrome." It is true that during the first year of daycare, kids have more coughs and colds than those who stay at home. However, research shows that after the first year the risk of infection is no different than that of the child kept at home. In fact, the child's defense mechanism "builds muscles" at the daycare "gym." Kids exposed early to daycare viruses tend to have fewer colds as they grow up than kids who were not exposed.

Myth: My doctor prescribed antibiotics because she wants to make sure I don't get pneumonia.

Facts: Your doctor probably prescribed antibiotics because she felt she had to do something for your cold and she didn't have anything better. You can help by not requesting antibiotics from your doctor. You could even give a copy of this book to your doctor! or maybe to the nurse in your doctor's office. In my experience, nurses are avid readers.

As you know by now, the great majority of acute coughs associated with colds and flu are due to viruses. Dr. William Schaffner, chairman of the department of preventive medicine at Vanderbilt University's School of Medicine in Nashville, said in an interview with WebMD, "Viral infections like the flu aren't affected by antibiotics." He continues, "You might as well take a placebo."

However, these antibiotics are not a simple sugar pill-placebo. They are potent drugs with dangerous side effects. Antibiotics should never be prescribed as a preventive treatment. You know, the "just in case" method! This was actually proven in a 1997 landmark study published in the prestigious *Journal of the American Medical Association*. The World Health Organization's acute cough recommendations state that antibiotics DO NOT prevent pneumonia.

Myth: I need a combination product for my cough — an expectorant and a cough suppressant — to cover all my bases.

Facts: As we have discussed throughout the book, OTC combination products are not only ineffective but they are dangerous. Most of the respected medical organizations and cough authorities have recommended for years that these products should be taken off the market — but the industry has rendered a deaf ear. So what can we do? STOP buying them NOW!

Myth: I have green mucus, which means I have bronchitis; I probably need antibiotics.

Facts: The mucus in acute viral respiratory infections has two phases. Initially, the mucus is clear and thin, layering the nose, back of the throat, sinuses and lungs. This phase usually lasts one to three days. Subsequently the mucus becomes thick and often turns yellow or green. This is absolutely normal. You don't need antibiotics.

Sometimes a secondary bacterial infection follows the initial viral infection. These secondary bacterial infections have a constellation of symptoms accompanying the green mucus. Usually the green mucus is associated with worsening of the cough, tiredness, low grade fever or fever and chills. Patients usually tell their doctors, "I was getting better from a cold (or a flu) that I have had for a week. But now I feel worse." That's key: if you are getting better and suddenly all the symptoms "feel worse"—secondary bacterial infection is likely the cause.

But remember, viral infections also produce green mucus, just like bacterial infections. So the green mucus by itself does not mean you have a bacterial infection which requires antibiotics. Check your other symptoms as well.

Now that you know the answers to the most common myths, let's move on to explore the world of chronic cough (a cough that lasts for more than four to six weeks). You'd be surprised, most of the time these coughs are both avoidable and treatable. But before we move on, I invite you to visit our website and post your questions so we can give you the facts! Please post questions of general interest as I am not able to address individual health conditions.

❧ ELEVEN ❧

Chronic Hackers
and the Art of Medicine

*"Code blue! Code blue! Room 7—Outpatient Pulmonary,"
came in loud and clear from the overhead while I was walking to
my office on a particularly busy Monday at the Cleveland Clinic
Florida Cough Center. "Respiratory arrest in outpatient—that's
unusual!" I thought to myself in the elevator. If people are having
a life-threatening asthma attack they go right to the emergency
room; they don't sit and wait in the outpatient clinic. And when
a code is called in a hospital—summoning a special emergency
team for a patient who suddenly seems to be at risk of dying—it's
usually for a heart attack, not a respiratory problem. In any case
I ran to the rescue. When I arrived, the room was full of nurses
and spectators and a jumble of orders.*

"Does she have a pulse?"

"Check the blood pressure!"

"Put oxygen on!"

"What's her O_2 sat [oxygen saturation level]?"

*Then suddenly, "She's awake, she's awake!" my nurse Darlene
exclaimed to me. "This is your new patient, Maria. She went into
a major coughing attack that left her speechless. Then she turned
blue and fell to the floor."*

This may sound dramatic but it's a true story. Maria's "cough attack" left her without air, creating what we call a "cough induced syncope" or fainting fit. She told me she had suffered from a persistent dry cough for twelve years and it was making her life miserable. She had even quit her job the year before, because she got tired of hearing her boss and co-workers complain of her cough. "Estas tuberculosa," they would say in Spanish— "You have tuberculosis." She heard this so many times that she started to believe she had something contagious. She went to countless doctors and specialists. She even went back to Cuba to see her doctor, but to no avail.

"This month alone, I've visited the doctors in the ER and urgent care clinics seven times. I get a Z-Pak or new antibiotic and prednisone every time I go. I'm a victim of the Z-Pak clinics, as you called them in that USA Today *interview. That's how I found you."*

She had been told that she had asthma, but I wanted to do my own examination to find the cause, whether a transient clinical condition or an underlying disease process. Only if I understand the underlying cause can I target a specific treatment.

I reviewed all her X-rays, CT scans, blood tests, and breathing tests and found no significant evidence to support the diagnosis of asthma. After using a laryngoscope (a flexible tube with a camera at the tip) to explore her nose, throat, and vocal cords, I told her she had severe gastric reflux. Her cough came from her stomach acid causing a spasm in her throat (laryngeal spasm).

The steroids she was taking for her misdiagnosis of asthma produced severe gastritis and made the reflux worse. Even more disturbing, the steroids caused her to gain more than 100 pounds in less than two years. She was astonished and confused that the drugs prescribed for her not only did not help, they had affected her negatively in many ways, including her self-esteem, her ability to exercise, and even the expense of buying a new wardrobe.

A week later I got a call from the ER—Maria was having another cough attack. I ran to the ER between patients to see her and treated her without steroids. Instead I taught her some breathing exercises, talked about diet, and used an antacid and some inhalers. She recovered without problems.

She came to my office for a followup visit determined to follow my instructions. It was a long journey of lifestyle changes—diet, exercise, and breathing exercises—but she was already feeling 80 percent better after only four weeks.

The cough that just won't go away

Chronic cough (a cough lasting more than four to six weeks) is a common and disturbing symptom that keeps many people trapped in embarrassment. If this is you, please seek the attention of an expert physician who understands that cough is a symptom with multiple causes. The role of the expert is to find the appropriate diagnosis and treatment. This chapter is not intended to be used for self-diagnosis or treatment. It is an educational tool that you can share with your doctor and contribute to finding your "Cough Cure."

We are not going to discuss infectious causes of chronic coughs like tuberculosis and fungal infections, because they usually run an aggressive course. This type of cough comes with a constellation of symptoms— such as fever, chills, mucus production, tiredness and general sense of being really sick—and it does require medical intervention.

We are going to explore reasons for cough in which you don't have the sense of being acutely sick. This is what I call "antisocial cough." This is not the "social cough" your mom used to interrupt inappropriate conversations. This is the cough that prevents you for going to movies, restaurants and social activities. This is the cough that drops your productivity and keeps you from enjoying life.

I've had the privilege of treating people with infectious and noninfectious coughs for over twenty years. I spent two years researching and treating infectious cough such as tuberculosis (still one of the most common causes of death worldwide) and many others during my research time in Venezuela's Orinoco River region.

The art of medicine

Before I dive into this fascinating topic, I need to make a clarification. Medicine is an art; medicine is not an exact science. It's not two plus two. In medicine, many times two plus two may equal 10. Why do I say this? Because some infections can stick to your lungs for months and even years without causing symptoms like fever, chills, and generalized malaise. Nontuberculous mycobacterias are the perfect examples. These families of mycobacterias are not contagious like tuberculosis. They love humidity and for some reason ladies as well! So when I see a chronic cough in a woman who lives in a humid climate (and especially, for some reason, a thin older woman) I know I need to screen for this type of mycobacteria.

So, to simplify the conundrum of chronic coughs without a clear infectious diagnosis, I'm going to use the algorithm I published in the *Cleveland Clinic Journal of Medicine* entitled "Q: How Should One Investigate a Chronic Cough?"

Once your doctor has gathered the full descriptive history of the cough and the associated symptoms; the first step in making the diagnosis is to obtain a chest X-ray (which your doctor will abbreviate "CXR"). If you have a chronic cough, you probably already have several chest X-rays or even a CT scan. Today in most ERs and doctors' offices, a chest X-ray or CT scan is done before even talking with the patient.

First do no harm: avoid unnecessary X-rays

While I am recommending a chest X-ray for *chronic (longterm)* cough, it is not recommended for an *acute (recent)* cough except under specific circumstances. I visited a large clinic recently in which every single patient was given a chest X-ray before seeing a doctor. Our oath as physicians is "First do no harm," but we are endangering our patients with this overuse of radiation. Doctors need to learn not to order unnecessary X-rays, and in the meantime, patients need to take responsibility for their own health. My dear friends, you need to be pro-active and ask your physician, respectfully, whether an X-ray is really necessary. Bring this book with you so you can share the guidelines on page 170.

How to investigate a chronic cough

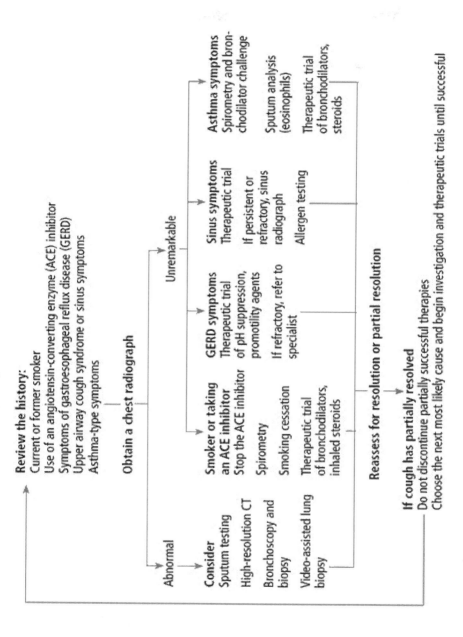

Review the history:
Current or former smoker
Use of an angiotensin-converting enzyme (ACE) inhibitor
Symptoms of gastroesophageal reflux disease (GERD)
Upper airway cough syndrome or sinus symptoms
Asthma-type symptoms

Obtain a chest radiograph

Abnormal

Consider
Sputum testing
High-resolution CT
Bronchoscopy and biopsy
Video-assisted lung biopsy

Unremarkable

Smoker or taking an ACE inhibitor
Stop the ACE inhibitor
Spirometry
Smoking cessation
Therapeutic trial of bronchodilators, inhaled steroids

GERD symptoms
Therapeutic trial of pH suppression, promotility agents
If refractory, refer to specialist

Sinus symptoms
Therapeutic trial
If persistent or refractory, sinus radiograph
Allergen testing

Asthma symptoms
Spirometry and bronchodilator challenge
Sputum analysis (eosinophils)
Therapeutic trial of bronchodilators, steroids

Reassess for resolution or partial resolution

If cough has partially resolved
Do not discontinue partially successful therapies
Choose the next most likely cause and begin investigation and therapeutic trials until successful

A chest X-ray is NOT necessary for an acute cough UNLESS one or more of these symptoms is present:

- persistent fever lasting more than four days,
- chills with shaking,
- more and more green or yellow secretions,
- coughing up blood,
- wheezing or significant shortness of breath, or
- chest pain with cough or deep breaths.

We doctors need to listen more

Physicians under time pressure have stopped doing a thorough interview, relying on diagnostic tests instead. But nothing can substitute for really listening to our patients. When I went to medical school in Cuba, we spent an entire year learning how to glean diagnostic information from interviewing our patients. (It was an indirect benefit from our lack of diagnostic equipment.) I find that 80 percent of diagnosis depends on taking a good patient history. I am blessed with the ability to help patients where other fine physicians have failed only because I delve so deeply with my questions.

Incomplete history—when doctors fail to gather all the information they could by really listening and paying attention to their patients—is without a doubt the greatest loss in the art of medicine. Incomplete history can cost you significant amounts of time and money spent on doctors and consultants. Incomplete history accounts for inappropriate tests and hospitalization costing millions in taxpayers' dollars each year. Even more disturbing is the fact that incomplete history contributes to the medical errors that result in hundreds of thousands of patient deaths per year (making medical errors the third leading cause of death in the United States).

It is for this reason that you should familiarize yourself with the key questions to ask your doctor in order to help make an accurate diagnosis of your cough. It will definitely save you money and time.

Years ago a colleague of mine came to my clinic suffering from a dry cough for two months. No other symptoms. He was healthy and in good physical shape. He was very concerned with radiation exposure, so it took me more than half an hour to convince him to get a chest X-ray. He knew I was very concerned with the overuse of chest X-rays and CT scans as well. (This was well-documented in a research study presented at the CHEST conference in 2015.)

We agreed on a simple chest X-ray that revealed a mass in his right lung. I went through the emotions of giving unpleasant news to a patient—even more so, to a friend. It looked like he had lung cancer, but to be absolutely sure, I went in and performed a bronchoscopy (a procedure in which I use a flexible thin tube with a camera at the tip). Going through the nose into the lungs, this incredible procedure allowed me to take samples for culture and biopsy.

The mass turned out to be fungus that grew in his lungs. He most likely got it from his regular trips to Phoenix, Arizona.

Arizona? Yes, the fungus *Coccidioides immitis* loves the dry heat of Arizona. Its tiny seed-like spores become wind-borne and get into your lungs. Fortunately, more than 60 percent of the people exposed to this "Cocci" will not develop an infection. Of those that do, most have no symptoms although they have changes that show up on an X-ray. Only a small percentage develop an active infection—we call it Cocci Valley Fever—with all of the symptoms of pneumonia. So it is very important to mention to your doctor any potential exposure to unusual microbes through travel.

Seek and you shall find—what doctors should look for

In addition to reporting travel exposure, tell your doctor about aerosolized chemicals, allergens, and any other substances that might have gotten into your lungs. Report any exposure to fumes, gas, vapors or dust in large quantities or for a prolonged period of time. Smoking is still the number one reason for chronic cough. Tell your doctor if you are on medications such as the family of angiotensin-converting enzymes (ACE) inhibitors (lisinopril, ramipril and other drugs whose generic names end in "-pril"), because they can cause a chronic cough.

Also report using the over-the-counter nasal spray Afrin (oxymetazoline). Afrin opens up the nasal passages but they close up as soon as the medication wears off. In fact the rebound effect makes your symptoms worse and worse. They come back even stronger, you keep using Afrin, the time lapse to the rebound gets shorter and shorter, then you need more and more. You have to use it to the point of burning your nose passages, creating a condition called "rhinitis medicamentosa." This fancy term, simply meaning "nose irritation caused by medicine," is a common reason for a chronic cough.

If a potential irritant is present, it should be avoided or stopped immediately. If the cough improves partially or fully when exposure to the irritant is stopped, this supports a diagnosis of bronchitis (inflammation of the windpipe).

The Bridge Zone, land of the recalcitrant cough

If something abnormal shows up on the chest X-ray, then this abnormality should guide the diagnostic inquiry. But if the chest X-ray is normal, then the cause most likely comes from area of our body I call the "Bridge Zone." This is the unclaimed territory at the back of the nose and throat, behind the tongue, in the vocal cords, and even in the upper part of the windpipe. This is the area where chronic recalcitrant cough often originates. ("Recalcitrant" usually refers to obstinately uncooperative kids. It's also a term that doctors use for a condition that stubbornly resists treatment. It's as though the cough has a mind of its own!)

The specialties that touch this area of our body only claim diseases that require surgery or a procedure. A cough coming from this area is an orphan, ignored by dentists, ear-nose-and-throat specialists, pulmonologists or gastroenterologists. Think about the names given to these specialties: the dentist must be responsible for just the teeth; the ear-nose-and-throat doctor—just that; the pulmonologist for just the lungs; and the gastroenterologist for the stomach. But who works on the diseases coming from the Bridge Zone? Some people want to call them "aerodigestive diseases" and create yet another new specialty. I believe that we need to resist the overspecialization of medicine. We all need to become better clinicians — doctors with critical thinking.

Chronic recalcitrant coughs coming from the Bridge Zone include conditions such as upper airway cough syndrome, postnasal drip, cough-variant asthma, exercise-induced asthma, gastroesophageal reflux disease (GERD) and neurogenic cough.

It is important to know that Bridge Zone coughs overlap most of the time. These are a few that overlap:

- ∾ true asthma made worse by reflux,
- ∾ postnasal drip made worse by reflux,
- ∾ reflux mimicking asthma, and
- ∾ postnasal drip mimicking shortness of breath or chest pain.

So the clinician treating a patient with chronic cough must differentiate, for example, between a cough *caused by* postnasal drip that gets *worse* from reflux versus a cough that *looks like* asthma but is *caused by* reflux. In the first case the primary treatment is aimed at stopping the postnasal drip, while in the second case the primary treatment is aimed at stopping the reflux.

This is what I mean by critical thinking and the Art of Medicine. No matter how many chest X-rays or CT scans the patient receives, the physician must still use her or his critical thinking to differentiate among possible causes. And it is this thought process — not all the diagnostic imaging — that will determine a course of treatment likely to actually stop the cough.

Testing, testing 1, 2, 3

Investigating chronic recalcitrant cough in most cases will require a laryngoscopy using a very thin flexible tube with a camera at the tip. This procedure allows the exploratory visualization of the Bridge Zone. Other procedures to explore the esophagus or food pipe may be necessary, as well as breathing tests to examine the lung capacity and a simple breath test to help us find asthma-like inflammation of the windpipe.

Neurogenic cough: the diagnosis of last resort

If all these tests are normal and do not point toward any specific cause, **neurogenic cough** is the most likely cause. This is a persistent dry cough, usually for years with no clear evidence of reflux or rhinosinus (nose and sinus) problems. This type of cough has received multiple names—neurogenic cough, hypersensitivity cough syndrome, chronic recalcitrant cough—but they all mean the same. Acid reflux can trigger this cough but it is not the main trigger. Some people develop it after a viral infection, others get it from environmental irritants—fumes, gas, fragrances, cleaning products.

It is called a neurogenic cough (meaning starting from the nerves) because the problem arises from irritated nerves in the cough receptors, areas in the throat and windpipe that sense mucus or allergens and tell the body to cough them out. These cough receptors are there to protect you, but sometimes they misfire or misperceive the problem. For example, acid reflux can irritate the nerves, but coughing won't help to clear out acid reflux. Nor will it clear out the vapors from fragrances, gas and cleaning products.

There are many reasons for this type of cough, one of the most common referrals to a cough expert. It is usually treated with medications for nerve problems such as gabapentin, amitriptyline and others. (If you are on one of these medications, tell your doctor when the cough is gone so that the medication can be discontinued.) On many occasions acid reflux treatment should also be addressed (see our recommendations on page 181).

Back to Buteyko breathing for chronic coughs

The Buteyko method described on page 96 was designed to help asthmatics and others with serious chronic breathing problems. It begins with a simple measurement exercise called a "control pause" that anyone can do at home. It's an estimate of how big you breathe, or your CO_2 level. It simply means testing how many seconds you can comfortably hold your breath after a normal exhalation. To do it accurately, you have to follow specific instructions, beginning with resting for several minutes (until your breathing is at baseline) before measuring.

- Take a small, silent breath in through your nose and allow a small silent breath out through your nose.
- Keep your mouth closed and hold your nose with your fingers to prevent air from entering your lungs.
- Count the number of seconds until you feel the first definite desire to breathe.
- At the first definite desire to breathe in, you may also feel the first involuntary movements of your breathing muscles. Your tummy may jerk or your throat may contract.
- Release your nose and breathe in through it.

Your inhalation at the end of holding your breath should be calm. If you are gulping for air, you held your breath too long. This is not a contest to see how long you can hold your breath! It's important to hold your breath only until you feel the first involuntary movements of your breathing muscles, or the first stress of your body telling you to "breathe."

The number of seconds of your "control pause" indicates how healthy your breathing is (40 to 60 seconds or more is considered healthy) or how unhealthy (less than 10, you're in trouble). Slight dysfunction can be corrected by learning about the method from a book or online, for example from the books (specific ones for asthma, anxiety, athletes and so forth) and videos by Patrick McKeown, an internationally prominent Buteyko teacher. Short clips from his videos are available on YouTube, and an extensive video interview is available at www.drmercola.com.

However, those with more severe dysfunction and especially those on medications need individualized instruction from a qualified Buteyko educator (www.buteykoeducators.org). Hadas Golan, the Buteyko educator at Boston Medical Center whom we met on page 96, frequently sees patients who have tried to learn the approach unsuccessfully from a book or online. The most common problem, she says, is that people try to force themselves to hold their breath too long, or they develop too much tension and their symptoms get worse because they've been trying to restrict their breathing too much.

If your cough is mild, you may be able to resolve it with this information alone. The more complicated your health history, and the more severe your symptoms, the more likely you are to need professional help.

Everyone can benefit from relaxed, gentle nasal breathing (if you can do it comfortably and make it your normal way of breathing). However, many people find it stressful and need more guidance. This is especially true for people with anxiety, because you may become more anxious if you feel as though you are breathing less.

People with a long history of asthma and other serious conditions typically have developed a dysfunctional breathing pattern that will take more guidance and practice than this simple advice. Generally if you have access to a Buteyko educator (one who works locally or by Skype), that's the best way to learn. Second best would be a book or DVD, just as with learning yoga. Just keep in mind Golan's tips about not restricting your breathing too much and not forcing yourself to hold your breath too long.

Spicy! — acid reflux cough

Acid reflux is probably one of the most common reasons for cough, throat irritation and even lung damage (lung fibrosis or scar tissue in the lungs) as it goes back down into the lungs through the vocal cords. Most people (and most doctors) think that the solution is antacids such as Tums, or proton pump inhibitors such Prilosec or Nexium.

Acid reflux actually has several causes and different possible solutions.

The symptoms come from stomach acid flowing in the wrong direction, up into the esophagus. That much we can agree on, and it's a serious problem. The stomach secretes acid in part to digest protein, but the stomach and esophagus muscles are made of protein. The stomach itself is protected by a layer of mucus so it doesn't digest itself, but the esophagus lacks this layer. So why isn't the esophagus digested as part of normal digestion?

The answer lies in a ring of muscles, like a drawstring, between the stomach and esophagus. This "lower esophageal sphincter" loosens when you swallow to allow food to pass into the stomach. Then it should tighten—but many factors in our lifestyle make it too relaxed, including:

- smoking and drinking alcohol;
- mint, chocolate, and caffeine;
- increased abdominal pressure from obesity or pregnancy;
- the hormones of pregnancy; and
- a long list of drugs, including antihistamines, muscle relaxants, and medications for asthma, high blood pressure, heart conditions, anxiety, depression, migraines, and diarrhea.

Stress can cause heartburn; stress reduction techniques such as meditation may be able to relieve it without drugs. Many people report the *symptoms* of acid reflux even though *tests* show that they do not have much acid in their esophagus. Research shows that stress may be increasing their *perception* of acid reflux but not the actual reflux.

In addition, holistic practitioners find that many of us as we age have *too little* in the way of digestive enzymes, including stomach acid. When there's not enough stomach acid, our food doesn't digest; instead it ferments in the stomach, and the "drawstring" does not get the signal to close as it normally would. With the drawstring open, acid can get up into the esophagus, even if there's not enough of it for efficient digestion.

Food allergies can be a problem; if you have reason to suspect food allergies, work with an integrative medicine doctor or naturopath (see Appendix B). These professionals can also help you safely reduce or even eliminate any medications causing acid reflux by using natural supplements and lifestyle changes. Acupuncture can be helpful; in one study, it worked better than doubling the patients' PPIs. Finally, the muscles in the stomach and the esophagus "drawstring" can become sluggish for many reasons, including diabetes, which is so widespread in our society, it can be a significant contributor to acid reflux.

Many of these factors, like diabetes, would be hard to treat, but either low or high stomach acid are relatively easy to treat. How can you tell which one? The simplest and safest approach is to treat yourself for low stomach acid and see if your symptoms get better. Try a teaspoon of apple cider vinegar in a little water before each protein-containing meal (it will taste like tart apple juice). Apple cider vinegar is one of the most widely used herbal remedies, with dozens of uses from arthritis to weight loss, as long as you get the brown unfiltered natural kind.

Or take a capsule of betaine hydrochloride (basically the same substance your stomach uses for digestion, in a capsule that makes it safe to swallow). My coauthor finds that many of her clients' acid reflux symptoms improve by *enhancing* stomach acid with one of these methods.

You could try it the other way around — using an antacid to treat yourself for *too much* stomach acid — but here's why we don't recommend starting with that (unless your doctor has diagnosed you with Barrett's esophagus or other serious condition caused by too much stomach acid). Your stomach secretes acid for several reasons, and research shows that blocking your normal, natural stomach acid can have serious consequences for your health:

- ✷ Stomach acid helps digest protein; suppressing it can contribute to muscle wasting and weakness in older people.
- ✷ It helps the body absorb minerals; suppressing it can contribute to osteoporosis, bone fractures, and a dangerous lack of magnesium, which is essential for healthy heart function.
- ✷ It is your body's first line of defense to kill parasites, viruses and other pathogens coming into your body and thereby prevent food-borne illnesses and others such as "C-diff" (the bug that causes terrible diarrhea). In an animal study, it even worked against prions like those that cause "mad cow disease."

- Stomach acid is how the body would normally kill the helicobacter organisms that cause stomach ulcers, so limiting stomach acid allows helicobacter to flourish.
- It's needed to release B_{12} from our food, so that limiting stomach acid can lead to a B_{12} deficiency.
- It's needed to enhance the bioavailability (effectiveness) of the vitamin C you get from food.

Finally, if you decide to stop the major antacids like Prilosec or Nexium (the drugs known as proton pump inhibitors or PPIs), the resulting rebound acid can be worse than what you started with. It's much safer and wiser to start your self-test with apple cider vinegar or betaine hydrochloride. Betaine hydrochloride (HCl) can cause a burning sensation if you are in fact too high in stomach acid, so before you take it prepare half a teaspoon of baking soda mixed in a glass of water in case you experience burning after the HCl supplement.

And if you conclude that you really do have too much stomach acid, there is a simple and harmless solution: drink more water, which dilutes the acid. In a research study that compared the effect on stomach acidity of drinking water to that of five different acid-blocking drugs, the water reduced stomach acidity in only one minute, while the drugs took up to 175 minutes to have the same effect. Note that for people who have *too little* stomach acid, it's important to avoid drinking water with meals so that you don't dilute your digestive juices.

Here's a little-known tip for heartburn-provoked coughs: Heartburn Free from Enzymatic Therapy, one of the best quality supplement companies. One box can keep you heartburn-free for several months. That's astounding for 10 doses of an herb (orange peel extract) that reduces acid *reflux* without reducing the stomach acid you *need* to digest your food. Also from Enzymatic Therapy: DGL Licorice, a safe form of licorice that not only works for heartburn, it helps with ulcers as well. Chew a couple of tablets half an hour before meals. Licorice is also one of the active ingredients in Gutsy Chewy, which also contains papaya, apple cider vinegar and xylitol, all well-researched supplements for oral and digestive health.

Here's another natural option: an algae-based foam that forms a sort of "raft" floating at the top of your stomach's digestive juices. This "raft" forms a barrier at the top of your stomach that prevents the acid from flowing up into the esophagus, instead keeping it in your stomach to digest your food. Life Extension's Esophageal Guardian provides the algae in berry-flavored chewable tablets; don't worry, they don't taste like seaweed! I'm giving you several options because different things work for different people.

Simple breathing exercises can provide another non-drug way to resolve acid reflux. Remember the ring of muscles at the top of your stomach, the one that's supposed to keep acid in your stomach where it belongs? And remember that the mischief may be caused by these muscles getting weak and saggy? This ring of muscles (called a sphincter) is surrounded by the diaphragm, the big, powerful sheet of muscle that causes you to breathe and cough. Research shows that your diaphragm muscles can be trained so that their strength helps contract your sphincter muscles.

In the bigger picture, how can we shift our digestive picture so we don't need to treat it on a day-to-day basis? Reflux is problem of the last 200 years. The number of people suffering from reflux keeps growing. It is not the lack of Tums or the "purple pill." It's a problem that came with our modern lifestyle.

Prior to the Industrial Revolution most people ate two meals a day, beginning with a large breakfast. Then they spent the whole day in the fields sweating and had dinner/supper at the end of the day. Since the Industrial Revolution and the invention of electricity, most people work indoors at sedentary jobs, TV was invented and later the Internet, "propaganda" in the form of advertising was born, and we were told we need to eat three or four or six times a day. As a result, America is the country with the highest number of diets published in the world!

Back to the 1700s to fix your reflux

If you suffer from reflux do the following:

How to Prevent and Treat Acid Reflux

- ∾ Try not to eat after 6 p.m.
- ∾ Allow more than three hours of digestion prior to going to sleep.
- ∾ Prop up your head with a pillow instead of lying flat in bed.
- ∾ Diet: Modify your diet by gradually adding more greens and fruits, and your wholesome ethnic foods the way your grandma made them, except ...
- ∾ Eliminate the good Mexican spices, jalapeño, onion, garlic and tomatoes, plus citrus fruits and fatty foods.
- ∾ Avoid things that can relax the sphincter that keeps acid out of your esophagus (mint, chocolate, alcohol, tobacco).
- ∾ Drop coffee to one cup a day.
- ∾ Run from sodas—yes, all of them, even the ones that look great in the TV commercials.
- ∾ Learn to hold the mouth shut to the temptations of refined grains, particularly products made from white flour. When possible substitute the whole grain: for example, brown rice instead of white rice, whole wheat bread instead of white bread and so on. In my practice, I find that patients who stop using bleached white flour clear up their postnasal drip, allergic rhinosinusitis and asthma, because bleached flour is such a strong pro-inflammatory.
- ∾ If you still have acid reflux, try apple cider vinegar (a teaspoon diluted in a little water) or a betaine hydrochloride capsule before meals.
- ∾ If those do not work, try Life Extension's Esophageal Guardian; Gutsy Chewy; or Enzymatic Therapy's Heartburn Free or DGL Licorice (different products work for different people).

This doesn't mean that you can't enjoy the ethnic food of your ancestors. No, no, no! That's one reason most diets fail! They take you away from the foods you enjoy, the ones your grandma made for you, the ones "engraved in your heart." I recommend a Mediterranean diet, it's ideal. Always limit the portions and avoid fried foods; add healthy fruits and vegetables, salads, and juices with no sugar added. Choose local and organic produce as often as possible, and try not to microwave your food if at all possible. Prepare meals from scratch, avoid pre-packaged and processed foods and of course artificial ingredients. Drop the intake of foods and beverages that increase acid and eat a couple of times a day.

Yes, back to the 1700s to allow time for digestion. Your body needs time to process all the nutrients and to enjoy the industrious undertaking of the chemical process that takes place after eating. Don't be rigid. If you need more than that, drink an herbal tea, eat a fruit, drink water, walk, stretch, take a couple of deep breaths and enjoy life.

Drip, drip, drip—nose, throat and cough

Postnasal drip can be solely responsible for the cough, or it could be an add-on or overlap to reflux, asthma and bronchitis. The diagnosis and treatment of these groups of conditions require the eyes of a trained clinician. However, dietary modifications always help. Remember: reflux and postnasal drip overlap any other condition. Just follow the above diet instructions and while you wait for your doctor's appointment, you can curb your postnasal drip with one of my recommended antihistamines (Claritin, Allegra, Zyrtec, Benadryl) or a mucus-dissolving supplement (NAC, Mucostop or Wobenzym, see page 62).

Prepare for your appointment with your cough doctor

If you have a chronic cough, you can help your doctor find the correct diagnosis by bringing in a copy of the form on page 184.

And whatever your condition, you can help your doctor do the best possible job for you in the short amount of time allotted, by typing up a clear and concise paragraph about your current symptoms, possible reasons, medications you are on, and tests that have already been done with their results. Your doctor needs to know if a test was done and came back normal ("WNL" or "within normal limits") because it means a possible diagnosis has been ruled out and the test does not need to be repeated.

If your condition is chronic, *briefly* summarize its course (when/why it started, tests you've had, medications you've tried). A list of all your current medications is especially important because each physician may not be aware of medications prescribed by others.

Your Shortcut Guide to Chronic Cough Care

- ∾ Practice our recommended breathing exercises on pages 91 and 167.
- ∾ Follow our acid reflux guidelines on page 173.
- ∾ Stop all possible irritants: cigarettes, dust, fumes, vapors.
- ∾ If you do this for four to six weeks and you still have a cough (it's now a chronic cough), you need to see a doctor (pulmonologist or allergist) who understands the principles in this book.
- ∾ If you find no improvement after another six weeks, don't hesitate to go to a cough expert for a second opinion.
- ∾ Keep a copy of all your X-rays and CT scans. If they are normal, do not allow them to be repeated "just in case."
- ∾ There is a Cough Cure more than 98 percent of the time. Think about that! Doctors can't fix diabetes, hypertension or advanced cancer but cough has a solution!
- ∾ The number one reason for treatment failure is neglecting to adhere to the treatment recommendations. If this happens to you, don't give up — just do it again.
- ∾ Share this book with your doctor.

Take This Information to Your Doctor
If You Have a Chronic Cough

Check off any of these factors that apply to you. It will save time at your appointment and increase the chances that your doctor can find the cause of your cough.

__ Smoker? __ current __ past (from _____ to _____)
__ Cough following a viral infection
__ Use of Afrin (oxymetazoline)
__ Use of ACE inhibitors
    (Lisinopril, Ramipril, other "-pril" drugs)
__ Exposure to aerosolized chemicals
__ Exposure to fumes, gas, vapors or dust
__ Exposure to mold
__ Travel exposure to unfamiliar microbes
    or environmental factors
__ Exposure to fungus such as *Coccidioides*
    via travel to California or Arizona
__ Food allergies
__ Symptoms of acid reflux, including burning in the back of the throat, belching, nausea, hoarseness, and a bitter or sour taste coming up from your stomach. (Consider trying our remedies for acid reflux first; if they relieve your symptoms and your cough, you don't need to go to your doctor.)

TWELVE

Keep the Filter Clean!
Prevention

Let's talk about prevention—some natural ways to keep a cough from getting started in the first place. Remember that a cough can come from irritants such as pollution or cigarette smoke, from an infection, or from acid reflux.

Use a HEPA filter. This type of filter takes out the tiniest particles from the air, including dust, smoke and allergens. You can get a HEPA filter for a single room, such as the bedroom of an allergic child; or built into a vacuum cleaner; or even added to the heating/airconditioning system for your whole house. You can also get a tiny ionizing air filter to wear around your neck when the air outside tickles your cough! Check www.allergyasthmatech.com, a great resource for these and other products to help allergy sufferers.

Check for mold. If you tend to start coughing when your central air or heat go on, or if you cough in your house but not anywhere else, you may have mold growing in the ducts of your ventilation system. Or you may have mold growing in the drywall of your house or under the wall-to-wall carpeting if they've been soaked in a flood or by a leaky roof. Mold must be taken very seriously as a source of airborne illness and needs to be removed professionally by a mold remediation company. For more information about the dangers of mold and how to remove it, see the documentary *Moldy: The Toxic Mold Movie* (https://moldymovie.com.)

Keep your nose and throat from drying out. The moist lining of your nose and throat act as a barrier to the entry of microbes; it's the first line of defense of your immune system in these areas. In the winter, your heating system is probably drying out the air and therefore these protective barriers. Airplanes are even worse: the air in planes is both dry and cold, plus you're in close contact with the international germ pool. That's why people tend to get sick after a long international flight. On the plane, keep drinking water and suck on throat lozenges like Two Trees, Ricola, Olbas or Vogel (see pages 59–60). At home, use a humidifier to keep humidity levels at 40 percent to 50 percent. (This is tricky because mold can grow if the humidity remains too high.)

Don't smoke at all, and if you haven't been able to stop yet, definitely don't smoke in the same room or car with other people, especially kids. The second hand smoke is really dangerous for them.

There are many ways to stop smoking using holistic methods. Acupuncture and hypnosis can be especially effective. In keeping with our previous recommendation of acupressure for coughs, you can massage your own hands or ears to quell the craving. Mindfulness meditation can work too; also physical activity, a favorite recommendation of Dr. Gus!

St. John's wort, the well-known herb used for depression, can work to help stop smoking as well, although it interacts with certain drugs, so you should clear it with your doctor if you are on prescription medications. Rhodiola, another herb used for depression, can help stop smoking—plus research shows it also helps with anxiety, obsessive compulsive disorder and fatigue (talk about side *benefits!*). Wild oats (*Avena sativa*) herbal tincture is a helpful adjunct to overcome any addiction: a dropperful in a glass of water, several times a day.

The stop-smoking effectiveness of nicotine delivered via e-cigarettes is not yet clear at the time of this writing. Another type of vapor could be inhaled instead: the fumes from black pepper! This common kitchen spice even protects against lung cancer in several research studies. Research shows that black pepper oil reduces the craving for nicotine, alleviates anxiety, and provides satisfying sensory stimulations in the chest which replace the stimulation from nicotine.

Black pepper essential oil is available online and can be used in an aromatherapy diffuser; added to a bowl of boiling water for steam inhalation; or added to the liquid for e-cigarette vaping. (Apparently just a few drops in 10 ml of liquid will work effectively without damaging your atomizer.)

Homeopathy can be wonderfully supportive for any of these methods and it can also work well on its own. The quickest and simplest way to get the benefits of homeopathy is through a combination remedy, one that blends the homeopathic its withdrawal symptoms. Natra-Bio has a two-part Stop-It Smoking Kit with lozenges and tablets; Liddell's Nicotine Free comes in a spray form; both brands work well. As I explained in the previous section about combination remedies, if one brand does not work for you, it means that it does not contain your best-matching remedy, so instead of giving up on homeopathy, just try another brand.

To get the full benefit of homeopathy to help you stop smoking, go to a professional homeopath who can help find the deeper reason for your addiction. Just as Dr. Gus explained about finding the underlying reason for a chronic cough in order to treat it effectively, so too in these cases the underlying emotional state must be treated before the client can stop smoking.

Clients in my (Burke Lennihan's) practice who have difficulty stopping smoking know only too well the dangers of tobacco but they are unable to stop because they are using it for self-medication. My clients who have had the greatest difficulty stopping are the ones who have the worst underlying trauma.

Homeopathy is a powerful yet gentle way to release past emotional traumas without having to relive them. Once that happens, my clients are able to stop smoking, using the same techniques that had not worked for them in the past. (I should add that my clients are all women and are unusually highly educated, here in the Harvard community, so this observation may not be relevant in other practices.)

In the meantime, health care professionals might bear in mind that a patient might be smoking to calm their anxiety from an underlying emotional trauma. Then we can be compassionate rather than judgmental with patients who sincerely and repeatedly try to stop smoking and are unable to. We can encourage them to explore the possibility of underlying trauma or anxiety in their life, and to release it with an appropriate therapy.

Avoid toxins in your environment. Americans are surrounded by thousands of chemicals in our household cleaners, pesticides, bodycare products, cosmetics, pet care products, and other substances we use every day. We mistakenly assume that the government has checked the ingredients for safety, just as we assume it has checked over-the-counter medications. In fact many of our common household products contain chemicals known to cause cancer or birth defects. Other chemicals can cause sneezing, runny nose and coughing, as if the body knows they are toxic and wants to get rid of them.

Dr. Gus has seen hair stylists in his cough clinic with lung damage from breathing in the chemicals in hair products. One salon owner who suffered from COPD (chronic obstructive pulmonary disease) found great relief when he sold the salon and cut back to working just two days a week.

This just goes to show how chemicals in ordinary household products can affect our lungs. Of course you don't want to get to the point of lung damage, so you can start now to rid your house of toxic chemicals. An excellent resource for checking ingredients is Environmental Working Group's website, www.ewg.org. It has sections on its website for safe food and bodycare, clean air and water, non-toxic cleansers, and raising healthy children.

If you are the type of person who coughs or gets a headache or other symptoms from fumes, try the homeopathic medicine Phosphorus described on page 78.

Cultivate healthy habits of daily exercise and stress reduction practices such as yoga, meditation and calm breathing, like the Buteyko methods described on pages 96 and 175. Yoga can be so effective for those with breathing problems, a recent research study showed that it worked as well as standard pulmonary rehabilitation techniques for patients with chronic obstructive pulmonary disease (COPD). Patients liked doing yoga better than the standard exercises, and yoga was easier for those who had knee problems or other reasons they couldn't do cycling or treadmill exercises

Of course yoga is wonderful for stress reduction, which can help prevent or relieve your cough. Acid reflux can be made worse by stress, and yoga can help relieve it.

Avoid refined sugar and especially high-fructose corn syrup (read labels, they are everywhere), because sugar has an immediate negative effect on your immune system. Artificial sweeteners are just as bad, though! Avoid aspartame (Equal) and sucralose (Splenda) as well. You and your kids will enjoy natural sweeteners such as stevia, xylitol, agave, and small amounts of manuka honey or raw honey. You can also sweeten things with fruit juice or stewed dried fruits. You'll be pleasantly surprised and your kids will never know. My favorite natural sweetener (more expensive but totally worth it for anyone heading towards diabetes) is Planetary Formulas' EarthSweet (stevia plus herbs). Stevia has even been shown to help manage blood sugar levels for diabetics.

Dr. Gus's guidelines for healthy living

Dr. Gus has many years of experience in counseling his cough patients in how to have a healthier lifestyle. He has found that people need to start with something really simple that they enjoy, then expand from there. His guidelines for patients are on the next page.

Dr. Gus's Guidelines for Healthy Living

~ Exercise every day; 20 to 25 minutes of walking is enough to start. Gradually increase your pace and power, and run instead of walking if you can.

~ If you have knee problems and can't walk, exercise your arms with an arm exercise bike.*

~ Go outside, take deep breaths, breathe in the fresh air.

~ Use an elastic band to strengthen your chest and improve your posture: hold your arms overhead in a Y and push them back gently to open your chest.

~ Maintain good posture while sitting: sit upright, back straight, move your shoulders back.

~ For good posture while walking, let your arms fall to your side, palms forward, and rotate your thumbs outward. Good posture will open up your lungs and make your breathing easier.

Your Shortcut Guide to Prevention Guidelines

~ Stop smoking; while quitting, avoid smoking inside or around children.

~ Do breathing exercises or Buteyko daily. Consider yoga.

~ Use a HEPA filter to remove allergens from the air.

~ Check for mold in your house after a flood or ice dam; use propolis in a vaporizer until you can have mold removed.

~ Avoid toxins in your food, bodycare, cleaning and other household products: check them with Environmental Working Group's Skin Deep and Dirty Dozen lists, www.ewg.org.

~ Avoid sugars and artificial sweeteners; use raw agave, fruit juice, stevia or xylitol instead.

---

*Available online in a wide variety of styles and prices. See for example a useful comparison of the different models on www.theinsidetrainer.com.

ঙ THIRTEEN ঙ

Let's Help One Another:
The Let's Pass It Down Club

On a recent spring afternoon, two teenage sisters were at dance practice after school for the end-of-the-year performance. Throughout practice they noticed that their friend Julie couldn't stop coughing and blowing her nose. Embarrassed by her constant cough and the obvious drip, she left early and missed the next rehearsal.

The next day, the older sister called Julie to make sure she was OK. Julie was still not feeling well in spite of countless attempts with different medications. Concerned about her classmate's health (plus Julie was the lead dancer), the teenager remembered that her mom knew a lot about natural cough cures and suggested that Julie's mom call her mom for ideas.

That evening her mom told Julie's mom Marsha all about natural remedies and explained why the medications hadn't worked. Marsha learned many ways to help her daughter feel better by asking Julie about all her symptoms and offering her hot herbal tea, a massage with essential oils, and a sweet little homeopathic pill.

Julie always liked having her mom give her a back rub, so she especially enjoyed the massage with a fragrant blend of oils. Her mom also put a few drops in a diffuser near Julie's bed. The next morning Julie was already feeling better. Two days later

Julie was back at dance practice, and by the end of the week she was
ready for the big performance.

Julie was happy to return to her rehearsals. When asked how she
was feeling, she shared her mom's wonderful experience of finding
helpful guidance from another mom.

This incident and others like it were what started the Let's Pass It Down Club. The girls in this story are my daughters, Amanda and Lauren. You met them in the beginning of this book. They are older now—old enough to tell their friends about natural healing for coughs. Yes, even kids can join! The Let's Pass It Down Club was created to be a place where members can share as well as find remedies, ideas and resources for a better and healthier lifestyle.

Julie, their friend, is real although her name and the details of her story have been modified to protect her identity. Today Julie's mom looks forward to being a charter member of the LPD Club, not only to search for new ideas that other members post, but also to share her own new discoveries about using essential oils—her favorite new mother-daughter bonding experience.

It is my dream that we all pass our knowledge down to the next generation. My family has become passionate as well about sharing the things we have learned with everyone we come in contact with. Even my daughters now look for opportunities to share the effectiveness of homeopathic remedies with their friends!

I wish that my Grandma Juana had shared with me all her knowledge of the healing herbs in her backyard. I regret not learning more from her. I wish I had asked more questions, such as how she knew when to use tamarind leaves, or salvia, or romerillo. She is gone now, but I believe that she is smiling down on our efforts. I hope that from now on each generation will share their knowledge with the next. Let's Pass It Down! Come join us at our new website: www.coughcuresbook.com.

I hope that you have gleaned valuable information from this book — that we have answered questions you might have had, and inspired questions you didn't even know you should be asking. Please use and share this website, as well as the information and resources you've received here, with your friends, family and colleagues. I encourage you to take advantage of the evidence, research and the tools we have provided here, and take an active role in every aspect of your health.

Remember what we suggested at the beginning of this book? Let's all embrace the goal of reducing unnecessary antibiotics by learning and applying the principle in this book. Ask your friends to do the same. Share this book with your friends and offer it to your primary care doctor, your pediatrician, your pulmonologist. Give it to your employer, specifically the person concerned with controlling healthcare costs, and bring their attention to the cost savings in Appendix C.

A note to my fellow doctors:

As I stated in the beginning of this book, the danger of antibiotic-resistant diseases is very real and we are killing ourselves with the abuse of something that was designed to help us. We have to be honest about what works, and the limitations of a lot of the treatments and medications commonly prescribed. If doctors want to prescribe a placebo because they have nothing to offer for viral illnesses, antibiotics should not be the placebo. Even if my fellow physicians believe that our natural methods work only by the placebo effect, better to use a natural placebo that won't cause damage in the long run in the form of numerous side effects and a body immune to antibiotics.

We cannot dismiss the ways that have been passed down from generation to generation or discount the place that natural remedies should have in our pursuit of health. To be clear, I am in no way dismissing the value of modern medicine! As an Intensivist (intensive care specialist) myself, I see patients benefit every day from the breakthroughs of the amazing scientific and medical minds of our time, and I am aware that the Intensive Care Unit is not the place for an herbal tea.

But where we can, we should absolutely be taking advantage of the power of what nature has given us and the tried and true methods that are available to anyone who is open. I spent the majority of my medical career refusing to recognize the value of homeopathic remedies and herbal practices. I was trained by professors who did not believe in their efficacy and effectiveness due to lack of evidence. But in all honesty, there are many unproven controversial treatments in Western medicine that are culturally accepted by our professors and used today simply because there aren't any other alternatives in our conventional medical system.

I have since realized that the trusted remedies that have been successful for hundreds and even thousands of years are worth our attention and respect. Our goal should always be to provide every patient with the best, most effective, and well-informed care possible.

Let's embrace these methods and provide the best care for our patients, families and ourselves. You can suggest this book to your patients because you know you can rely on the soundness of the methods. I encourage my fellow physicians to contact me for CME courses based on this book at www.coughcuresbook.com.

I feel I have been blessed with this knowledge and I am grateful for the opportunity to share it with patients and physicians all over the country.

— Dr. Gus

Your Shortcut Guide to Natural Remedies

If you are new to natural healing and feel more comfortable in a drugstore than in a health food store, the best way to start is with the homeopathic cough syrups and combination remedies in a drugstore. They each have different remedies in the formula and each one has its fans. If one does not work for you, chances are another one will. You'll need to choose between a homeopathic cough syrup (the liquid will help soothe your throat) and pellets (easier to carry around):

- ∾ Chestal by Boiron,
- ∾ Hyland's Cough Syrup 4 Kids,
- ∾ Hyland's Cold 'n Cough Nighttime 4 Kids, or
- ∾ Cough & Bronchial Syrup by B&T (Boericke & Tafel).

Homeopathic remedies generally give quicker results than herbs, but perhaps you prefer a hot cup of herb tea or a fruit-flavored herbal cough syrup. Your grocery store may have these, or you can easily get any of these products online. A health food store will have a better selection and knowledgeable staff to guide you. Here's a start:

- ∾ Throat Coat Tea by Traditional Medicinals
  for a scratchy throat,
- ∾ Breathe Easy Tea to open up your airways,
- ∾ Elderberry antiviral syrup by Gaia (or any good brand), or
- ∾ Planetary Formulas Loquat Respiratory Syrup.

If you'd rather start with what you have in your kitchen:
- fresh-squeezed lemon juice in hot water
- honey
- garlic or ginger
- apple cider vinegar (dilute a little in water)
- salt water for a saline gargle or nasal flush
- dark chocolate
- chicken soup, preferably home made
- Vicks Vaporub for a foot rub.

And if you feel more confident buying a pharmaceutical, the only kinds Dr. Gus recommends are an antihistamine (Claritin, Allegra, Zyrtec, Benadryl) and a low dose of Tylenol (less than 1500 mg a day total and only when needed).

For nasal congestion:
- Xlear Nasal Spray with xylitol,
- NeilMed saline nasal rinse,
- a neti pot rinse, or, as a last resort,
- any saline nasal spray.

For acid reflux:
- Try apple cider vinegar (1 teaspoon diluted in a little water) or a betaine hydrochloride capsule before meals first.
- If they don't work, use Life Extension's Esophageal Guardian or Enzymatic Therapy's Heartburn Free or DGL Licorice.

❧ APPENDIX B ↬

Professional Treatment for Your Cough

If you have a persistent cough that does not respond to conventional or natural treatment after four to six weeks, or if it gets better then keeps coming back, you need to see your doctor for a full diagnostic workup. There is an outside chance that a persistent cough can be caused by lung cancer, even in a non-smoker. There are other potential conditions that can only be detected with the advanced diagnostic techniques of conventional medicine.

Once you have an accurate diagnosis, take your results to a local pulmonologist, allergist or ENT (ear, nose and throat doctor) who endorses the principles in this book, or who is willing to read it and follow its principles. Offer your physician a copy of this book with respect and appreciation for her or his medical knowledge.

If conventional medicine has no treatment for your condition, or if you prefer a natural approach, you may choose to work with a holistic physician, a naturopath or a homeopath. How to choose? This section is excerpted from Burke Lennihan's *Your Natural Medicine Cabinet.*

Holistic physicians are fully trained and licensed conventional doctors who prefer to work with supplements and natural medicines rather than with drugs. They may call themselves integrative medicine doctors or functional medicine doctors. Advantages include their knowledge of conventional medicine and their ability to monitor any necessary prescription medications.

On the other hand, these doctors are in great demand. Your community may not have any, or they may not be taking new patients. They often don't take insurance because they spend much more time with patients than insurance will cover. They may prescribe a lot of supplements, which are likely to be expensive and not covered by insurance. Their services are totally worth it if you can possibly afford them. You will most probably save a lifetime of co-pays and prescription drug expenses.

If you have a serious, potentially life-threatening illness, such a physician is recommended even if it involves traveling to another city and paying out of pocket. Bottom line: these physicians may not be easy to find, but they are well worth seeking out. Search these directories:

- http://www.abihm.org/search-doctors
- https://aihm.org
- https://www.functionalmedicine.org/practitioner_search. aspx?id=117

Naturopathic doctors (NDs rather than MDs) are usually easier to find and less expensive than holistic doctors yet they are comparable in their holistic training, provided they graduated from an accredited school.* You might choose based on insurance coverage, proximity, and word of mouth. Some states license naturopaths, others do not; in "licensed states," naturopathic care may be covered by insurance. Check licensed states here:

- http://www.naturopathic.org/content.asp?contentid=57

To find a naturopathic doctor near you, search the American Academy of Naturopathic Physicians:

- http://www.naturopathic.org/AF_MemberDirectory.asp? version=2

---

*The accredited schools of naturopathy are Bastyr, Boucher Institute, Canadian College of Naturopathic Medicine, National College, the National University of Health Sciences, Southwest College, and the University of Bridgeport. Beware of people calling themselves naturopaths based on online training.

As for a **professional homeopath,** homeopathy shines when there is a mind-body component to the chronic condition, or when it started after a specific event or exposure. Homeopaths call this the "Never Well Since," as in "I've never been the same since [an episode or trauma in your life]. " Here are a few ways you can tell whether homeopathy is likely to be your best option:

- ❧ If your cough is worse when you are under stress or experiencing a strong emotion such as anger or grief,
- ❧ if your chronic cough started at the same time you were going through a major trauma or stress, or
- ❧ if your chronic cough started when you were exposed to a particular allergen or toxin.

Professional homeopaths may or may not have a license in another health care modality. If your condition is serious, you either need to find a homeopath who is also medically licensed, or you need to be under the care of a physician willing to monitor your condition while you are pursuing a natural approach.

Homeopaths who are also medical doctors are listed in this directory:

- ❧ http://homeopathyusa.org/member-directory.html.

They generally do not take insurance because the homeopathic process takes too long for the amount of time that insurance will cover for an appointment. In case you can't find a medical-doctor-homeopath near you (there are fewer than 100 in the whole country), here are other options for finding a professional homeopath:

- ❧ www.homeopathicdirectory.org (nationally certified homeopaths)
- ❧ http://homeopathic.org/find-homeopath.

Both directories list any licenses in other health care modalities in addition to homeopathic credentials.

Sometimes the best homeopaths are not listed in directories. Homeopaths who have been in practice the longest, and homeopaths who are also medical doctors, may not list in directories because they already have such a long waiting list. That's why word of mouth is also a good option for finding a homeopath.

❧ APPENDIX C ❧

Saving Money
with the Best of Both Worlds

For people reading this book, it will help you save on co-pays for doctor's appointments and on drugs like antibiotics, tylenol and ibuprofen. Drugs for respiratory issues were the biggest category in the $40 billion that Americans spent for over-the-counter medications in 2015, accounting for $7.7 billion in sales, while painkillers were the fourth biggest category (nearly $4 billion).*

You can save on drugs in both categories after reading this book, because you may well be able to treat yourself at home and you won't even need an antibiotic or painkiller. You will learn how to understand those confusing labels on over-the-counter medications so you can choose the less expensive generic version (typically costing less than $10) and avoid potentially dangerous combination medicines that include drugs you don't need. Then you can choose the correct medication for your problem the first time around, avoiding countless return trips to pharmacy to try a different one. This will save you time as well as money.

If you want to go the natural route, homeopathic medicines are especially cost-effective because they work so quickly: one bottle typically costs less than $10 and is likely to last your family for a year or more.

*A reminder that research documentation for this and other statements in the book can be found in the Endnotes. Endnotes for this section start on page 256.

You probably won't use it up on a single cough or cold or flu. So the cost-savings compared to antibiotics becomes even greater.

You also need to consider the time you lose going to the doctor or taking your child to the pediatrician. Depending on your job, you may need to use up part of your sick leave or lose some of your pay.

There's an even bigger cost savings with natural methods. When you take an antibiotic, it makes you more likely to get sick again, because it undermines your immune system by destroying the friendly flora in your gut. Then you get into the vicious cycle that so many parents see with small children: the child gets sick, needs an antibiotic, gets sick again, back to the doctor again for another antibiotic and so on. When you use an herb or homeopathic medicine, it increases your overall health and immune system strength.

I (Burke Lennihan) can tell you about this from my practice in Cambridge, Mass., where Harvard and MIT attract families from all over the world. A family from Germany or India or South America might typically bring their children to see me because they want to establish a relationship with a homeopath for their children, just as they have back home.

I see these robust-looking children, with bright eyes and rosy cheeks, sitting quietly through an hour-long appointment, answering my questions clearly and respectfully—so different from typical American kids in my practice! The mothers will tell me, for example, "My child is the only one in his second-grade class who never has to stay home sick from school and has never been on an antibiotic, because I treat him at home with homeopathic remedies." We can teach American parents to do the same for their children, providing long-term cost savings and more importantly, a strong lifelong foundation for their children's health.

For corporations, treating acute illnesses quickly can provide immediate cost-savings beyond what has been possible to date with corporate wellness programs. These programs have been a great success in terms of employee satisfaction but somewhat of a disappointment in terms of return on investment (ROI), for a couple of reasons:

- ❧ The typical programs (yoga classes, lunchtime walking groups, gym memberships, better food choices in the cafeteria) are aimed at reducing chronic disease, but the payoff is likely to be years in the future rather than in the same fiscal year as the investment.
- ❧ A program like Dean Ornish's that can actually reverse heart disease involves a total immersion in exercise, stress reduction, yoga and an extreme change in diet; most corporate wellness programs are only able to offer a fraction of that radical change.

Providing incentives for employees to use the approach in this book could show an immediate change in absenteeism, presenteeism (employees showing up at work too sick to be productive), and the spread of contagious illnesses by employees who should have stayed home sick. If companies change the metric—benchmarking the cost of absenteeism and presenteeism in addition to health care premiums—they will see an immediate increase in savings and ROI for the wellness program.

There are additional benefits to employers from encouraging employees' medical self-care with our safe and effective methods:

- ❧ reduced insurance claims for primary care and emergency room visits and prescriptions for antibiotics
- ❧ greater motivation for employees to participate in more *long-term* lifestyle changes based on noting an *immediate* benefit from our recommendations (based on research studies), and
- ❧ reduced employee turnover resulting in reduced replacement costs; in one hospital, wellness programs focused on self-care, self-healing practices and lifestyle changes reduced employee turnover costs by $1.5 million in the first year.

The current corporate wellness offerings (typically yoga, exercise, healthy snacks in the vending machines) would still be important. The methods in this book could be added, with lunch-and-learn classes in topics like acupressure, breathing exercises, and natural methods to support smoking cessation.

For the health care system, the same type of savings will apply as in the corporate world.

Perhaps in the future the standard of care for each illness will include natural as well as pharmaceutical options. The Integrated Healthcare Policy Consortium (IHCP) has documented the value of holistic medicine's Therapeutic Order* in achieving the Triple Aim:**

- ✍ improving the patient experience of care (including quality and satisfaction)
- ✍ improving the health of populations
- ✍ reducing the per capita cost of care.

Washington state is like a laboratory for this model of health care, because for more than 20 years it has mandated coverage for *all* licensed healthcare providers, whether conventional or CAM (complementary and alternative medicine) professionals. Patients who used CAM in addition to conventional health care saved the system $367 a year (according to insurance claims data, after adjusting for demographic and health-related variables). In other words, although insurers and governments balk at covering holistic health care because of the so-called "additional costs," in fact it saves a substantial amount of money.

Physicians as well as patients would benefit from using our recommendations for acute viral illnesses as part of such a Therapeutic Order/

---

*Therapeutic Order—a term originally used by naturopathic physicians and now recognized as referring to holistic and traditional healing modalities in general—refers to the practice of using the lowest-force, least toxic, risky or invasive treatment first. Only if the first treatment fails are more risky or invasive treatments attempted, with drugs and then surgery the treatments of last resort.

**The concept of the Triple Aim was first introduced by the Institute for Healthcare Improvement's then President and CEO Donald Berwick, MD in an article he wrote in 2008. It became part of national healthcare policy two years later when Berwick left IHI to head the Centers for Medicare and Medicaid Services and announced the Triple Aim as "our highest-level goal." The following year the Agency for Healthcare Research and Quality incorporated the Triple Aim into its National Strategy for Quality Improvement in Health Care. Although none of these agencies specifically included holistic modalities in their strategies, the integrative healthcare professions turned out to be "a natural" for achieving the goals of the Triple Aim.

Triple Aim initiative. Primary care physicians and pediatricians today find it increasingly difficult to treat patients effectively because of short appointment times and patients who come back again and again with the same complaint. If these physicians are currently allotted only 15 minutes or so per patient; if most everyday complaints could be resolved at home with natural medicines; then these physicians could spend an hour per patient on the difficult cases that really need them, giving them greater job satisfaction while the health care system provides better results.

We return to a concept from the beginning of this book: other industrialized nations have better health care outcomes at a lower cost than the United States, and part of the difference is the inclusion of one or more natural healing modalities.

For a vision of how natural healing could play a greater role in U.S. health care, we recommend Dr. Len Saputo's *A Return to Healing* and Robert Duggan's *Breaking the Iron Triangle*. Both books include extensive documentation of the cost savings involved. For a dramatic, colorful and concise introduction to holistic modalities and the potential savings involved—backed by dozens of research studies—see the website of the Integrative Healthcare Policy Consortium, www.ihpc.org.

Modern medicine has provided powerful and readily available life-saving drugs, and Americans benefit from greater access to these drugs than people in developing countries like Cuba. Yet lack of knowledge about these drugs can lead to their misuse and undermine their effectiveness. We want to teach safe, effective and cost-effective medicines, both OTC and natural, while encouraging people to take more of an active role in partnering with healthcare professionals in the pursuit of good health.

❧ APPENDIX D ❧

Research Evidence for
Herbs and Supplements

Nearly all the herbs and supplements recommended in this book are supported by at least one research study. Some have dozens or even hundreds of studies; only three or four of those were cited here. Where possible, research on coughs or asthma was cited, otherwise we used at least one study indicating medicinal action. Research on homeopathy is covered in Appendix E and research on the effectiveness of natural methods (breathing exercises, acupressure) is covered in Appendix F.

American ginseng

McElhaney JE, Goel V et al. Efficacy of COLD-fX [American ginseng extract] in the prevention of respiratory symptoms in community-dwelling adults: a randomized, double-blinded, placebo controlled trial." *J Altern Complement Med.* 2006 Mar;12(2):153-7. PMID: 16566675. "Ingestion of COLD-fX by immunocompetent seniors ... reduced the relative risk and duration of respiratory symptoms by 48% and 55%, respectively."

McElhaney JE, Gravenstein S et al. A placebo-controlled trial of ... American ginseng to prevent acute respiratory illness [ARI] in institutionalized older adults. *J Am Geriatr Soc.* 2004 Jan;52(1):13-9. PMID: 14687309. "[American ginseng extract] was shown to be safe, well tolerated, and potentially effective for preventing ARI due to influenza and RSV ... 89% relative risk reduction."

Andrographis

Gabrielian ES, Shukarian AK et al. A double blind, placebo-controlled study of *Andrographis paniculata* fixed combination Kan Jang in the treatment of acute upper respiratory tract infections including sinusitis. *Phytomedicine* 2002 Oct;9(7):589-97. PMID: 12487322. "[Andrographis] has a positive effect in the treatment of acute upper respiratory tract infections and also relieves the inflammatory symptoms of sinusitis."

Saxena RC, Singh R et al. A randomized double blind placebo controlled clinical evaluation of extract of *Andrographis paniculata* (KalmCold) in patients with uncomplicated upper respiratory tract infection. *Phytomedicine* 2010 Mar;17(3-4):178-85. PMID: 20092985. "From day 3 to day 5 most of the symptoms in placebo treated group either remained unchanged (cough, headache and earache) or got aggravated (sore throat and sleep disturbance) whereas in KalmCold treated group all symptoms showed a decreasing trend." The andrographis extract was more than twice as effective as placebo.

Apple cider vinegar

Abe K, Kushibiki T et al. Generation of antitumor active neutral medium-sized alpha glycan in apple cider vinegar fermentation. *Biosci Biotechnol Biochem* 2007 Sep;71(9):2124-9. PMID 17827702. "The constituent neutral medium-sized alpha-glycan acts as an antitumor agent against experimental mouse tumors."

Balsam

Hedayat KM. Essential oil diffusion for the treatment of persistent oxygen dependence in a three-year-old child with restrictive lung disease with respiratory syncytial virus pneumonia. *Explore.* 2008;4(4):264-266. PMID: 18602620. "The [3-year-old] child had an 18-day history of oxygen requirement with acute desaturation episodes even while receiving high-flow oxygen and mucolytic therapy [for ten days in the hospital]. ... Balsam fir is reputed to have strong antimicrobial action, particularly with regard to pulmonary infections. ... Within 12 hours, oxygen requirement was reduced, blood oxygen saturation increased, and desaturation episodes abated. On the second day of oil use ... the child was weaned off the oxygen and discharged home. "

Berries

Adams LS, Kanaya N et al. Whole blueberry powder modulates the growth and metastasis of MDA-MB-231 triple negative breast tumors in nude mice. *J Nutr.* 2011 Oct;141(10):1805-12. PMID: 21880954. "Tumor volume was 75% lower in mice fed the 5% blueberry diet and 60% lower in mice fed the 10% blueberry diet than in control mice (P≤ 0.05)."

Krauze-Baranowska M, Majdan M et al. The antimicrobial activity of fruits from some cultivar varieties of *Rubus idaeus* and *Rubus occidentalis. Food Funct.* 2014 Oct;5(10):2536-41. PMID 25131001. "Two human pathogens *Corynebacterium diphtheriae* and *Moraxella catarrhalis* proved to be the most sensitive to raspberry extracts."

McAnulty LS, Nieman DC et al. Effect of blueberry ingestion on natural killer cell counts, oxidative stress, and inflammation prior to and after 2.5 h of running. *Appl Physiol Nutr Metab.* 2011 Dec ;36(6):976-84. PMID: 22111516. "Daily blueberry consumption for 6 weeks increases NK cell counts, and acute ingestion reduces oxidative stress and increases anti-inflammatory cytokines."

Rossi R, Serraino I et al. Protective effects of anthocyanins from blackberry in a rat model of acute lung inflammation. *Free Radic Res.* 2003 Aug;37(8):891-900. PMID: 14567449. "The anthocyanins contained in the blackberry extract exert multiple protective effects in carrageenan-induced pleurisy."

Black pepper (active ingredient piperine)

Lin Y, Xu J et al. Piperine induces apoptosis of lung cancer A549 cells via p53-dependent mitochondrial signaling pathway. *Tumour Biol.* 2014 Apr;35(4):3305-10. PMID: 24272201. "Piperine could be developed as an effective antitumor agent in the prevention and treatment of lung cancer without toxicity to the host."

Rose JE, Behm FM. Inhalation of vapor from black pepper extract reduces smoking withdrawal symptoms. *Drug Alcohol Depend.* 1994 Feb;34(3):225-9. PMID: 8033760. "Reported craving for cigarettes was significantly reduced in the pepper condition relative to each of the two control conditions [menthol and empty cartridge] ... negative affect and somatic symptoms of anxiety were alleviated in the pepper condition ... the intensity of sensations in the chest was also significantly higher for the pepper condition. These results support the view that respiratory tract sensations are important in alleviating smoking withdrawal symptoms."

Selvendiran K, Thirunavukkarasu C et al. Chemopreventive effect of piperine on mitochondrial TCA cycle and phase-I and glutathione-metabolizing enzymes in benzo(a)pyrene induced lung carcinogenesis in Swiss albino mice. *Mol Chem Biochem.* 2005 Mar;271(1-2):101-6. PMID: 15881660. "Piperine supplementation ... indicated an antitumour and anticancer effect."

Selvendiran K, Prince Vijeya Singh J, et al. In vivo effect of piperine on serum and tissue glycoprotein levels in benzo(a)pyrene induced lung carcinogenesis in Swiss albino mice. *Pulm Pharmacol Ther.* 2006;19(2):107-11. PMID 15975841. "Piperine was found to suppress benzo(a)pyrene (B(a)p) induced lung cancer in Swiss albino mice."

Black tea *see* Tea, green or black

Boswellia

Abdel-Tawab M, Werz O, Schubert-Zsilavecz M. *Boswellia serrata*: an overall assessment of in vitro, preclinical, pharmacokinetic and clinical data. *Clin Pharmacokinet.* 2011 Jun;50(6):349-69. PMID: 21553931. "Animal studies and pilot clinical trials support the potential of B. serrata gum resin extract (BSE) for the treatment of a variety of inflammatory diseases like inflammatory bowel disease, rheumatoid arthritis, osteoarthritis and asthma. ... In view of the results of clinical trials and the experimental data from in vitro studies of BSE, and the available pharmacokinetic and metabolic data on boswellic acids, this review ... underlines BSE as a promising alternative to NSAIDs."

Ferrara T, De Vincentiis G, Di Pierro F. Functional study on Boswellia phytosome as complementary intervention in asthmatic patients. *Eur Rev Med Pharmacol Sci.* 2015 Oct;19(19):3757-62. PMID: 26502867. "[Asthmatic] subjects receiving [purified Boswellia extract] 500 mg/day in addition to the standard treatment [inhaled corticosteroids and long-acting beta-agonists] showed a decrease in the number of inhalations needed compared to patients who did not receive [Boswellia] therapy. The treatment was well tolerated and only mild-moderate adverse events were registered."

Gupta I, Gupta V et al. Effects of *Boswellia serrata* gum resin in patients with bronchial asthma: results of a double-blind, placebo-controlled, 6-week clinical study. *Eur J Med Res.* 1998 Nov 17;3(11):511-4. PMID: 9810030. "70% of patients [treated with

Boswellia] showed improvement of disease as evident by disappearance of physical symptoms and signs such as dyspnoea, rhonchi, number of attacks, increase in FEV1, FVC and PEFR as well as decrease in eosinophilic count and ESR. ... Only 27% of patients in the control group showed improvement."

Butterbur

Danesch UC. *Petasites hybridus* (Butterbur root) extract in the treatment of asthma—an open trial. *Altern Med Rev.* 2004 Mar;9(1):54-62. PMID: 15005644. "The number, duration, and severity of asthma attacks decreased [on the *Petasites hybridus* extract Petalodex], while peak flow, forced expiratory volume (FEV1), and all measured symptoms improved during therapy. In addition, more than 40 percent of patients using asthma medications at baseline reduced intake of these medications by the end of the study."

Lee DK, Gray RD et al. A placebo-controlled evaluation of butterbur and fexofenadine [Allegra] on objective and subjective outcomes in perennial allergic rhinitis. *Clin Exp Allergy* 2004 Apr;34(4):646-9. PMID: 15080820. "Butterbur and fexofenadine, in comparison to placebo, were equally effective in attenuating the nasal response to AMP and in improving nasal symptoms, highlighting a potential role for BB in the treatment of allergic rhinitis."

Lee DK, Haggart K et al. Butterbur, a herbal remedy, confers complementary anti-inflammatory activity in asthmatic patients receiving inhaled corticosteroids. *Clin Exp Allergy.* 2004 Jan;34(1):110-4. PMID: 14720270. "Chronic dosing with BB [butterbur] conferred complementary anti-inflammatory activity in atopic asthmatic patients maintained on inhaled corticosteroids. Further studies are now required to assess the potential role for BB as either monotherapy in milder patients or add-on therapy in more severe asthmatics."

Schapowal A. Randomised controlled trial of butterbur and cetirizine [a non-sedating antihistamine] for treating seasonal allergic rhinitis. *British Medical Journal* 2002 Jan 19;324(7330):144-6. "Improvements in both the SF-36 and CGI (clinical global impression scale) were similar in both groups."

Camphor

Edris AE. Pharmaceutical and therapeutic potentials of essential oils and their individual volatile constituents: a review. *Phytother Res.* 2007 Apr;21(4):308-23. PMID: 17199238. "The possible role and mode of action of these natural products is discussed with regard to the prevention and treatment of cancer, cardiovascular diseases including atherosclerosis and thrombosis, as well as their bioactivity as antibacterial, antiviral, antioxidants and antidiabetic agents."

Hamidpour R, Hamidpour S et al. Camphor (*Cinnamonum camphora*), a traditional remedy with a history of treating several diseases. *Int J Case Reports Images* 2013;4(2):86–89. This literature review provides citations for research studies on camphor's effectiveness for a wide variety of diseases including cancer.

Cardamom

Majdalawieh AF, Carr RI. In vitro investigation of the potential immunomodulatory and anti-cancer activities of black pepper (Piper nigrum) and cardamom (Elettaria cardamomum). *J Med Food.* 2010 Apr;13(2):371-81. PMID: 20210607. "Our findings strongly suggest that black pepper and cardamom exert immunomodulatory roles and antitumor activities .... We anticipate that black pepper and cardamom constituents can be used as potential therapeutic tools to regulate inflammatory responses and prevent/attenuate carcinogenesis."

Catnip

Gilani AH, Shah AJ et al. Chemical composition and mechanisms underlying the spasmolytic and bronchodilatory properties of the essential oil of *Nepeta cataria L. J Ethnopharmacol.* 2009 Jan 30;121(3):405-11. PMID: 19041706. "*Nepeta cataria* possesses spasmolytic and myorelaxant activities mediated possibly through dual inhibition of calcium channels and PDE, which may explain its traditional use in colic, diarrhea, cough and asthma."

Nostro A, Cannatelli MA et al. The effect of *Nepeta cataria* extract on adherence and enzyme production of Staphylococcus aureus. *Int J Antimicrob Agents.* 2001 Dec;18(6):583-5. PMID: 11738350. "DNAse, thermonuclease and lipase were inhibited... a reduction of adherence was also observed."

Cayenne pepper

Baudoiin T, Kalogjera L, Hat J. Capsaicin significantly reduces sinonasal polyps. *Acta Otolaryngol.* 2000 Mar;120(2):307-11. PMID: 11603795. "Topical treatment with capsaicin significantly increased nose sinuses air volume and very significantly improved subjective and endoscopy scores, but did not significantly alter eosinophil cationic protein levels in nasal lavages."

Zhen C, Wang Z, Lacroix JS. Effect of intranasal treatment with capsaicin on the recurrence of polyps after polypectomy and ethmoidectomy. *Acta Otolaryngol.* 2000 Jan;120(1):62-6. PMID: 10779188 "These observations suggest that endoscopic surgery followed by intranasal capsaicin application reduces polyps and nasal obstruction recurrence and could be an alternative treatment to expensive corticosteroids in developing countries."

Cedar

Naser B, Bodinet C et al. *Thuja occidentalis* (Arbor vitae): a review of its pharmacological and clinical properties. *Evid Based Complement Altern Med.* 2005;2(1):69-78. . PMID: 15841280. "White cedar extracts stimulate an increase in spleen cell proliferation rates, cytokine induction, an increase in nitric oxide production, an increase in the number of antibody-producing lymphocytes, ... T-cell proliferation and increased differentiation into fully functional helper T-cells....In vivo study results also demonstrate [cedar's] immunopharmacological potential, including increases in white blood cells and cytokine induction, an increase of the antibody response in mice, short and long-term increases in the immune response of mice, and inhibition of influenza A virus pathology in mice."

Hauke W, Köhler G et al. Esberitox® N [a blend of white cedar, echinacea and wild indigo] as supportive therapy when providing standard antibiotic treatment in subjects with a severe bacterial infection (acute exacerbation of chronic bronchitis). A multicentric, prospective, double-blind, placebo-controlled study. *Chemotherapy*

2002;48(5):259-66. PMID: 12476043. "Patients received a new generation macrolide antibiotic ... together with either Esberitox® N ... or placebo ... The Esberitox group showed improvement in FEV1 more quickly than the placebo group."

Chamomile

Srivastava JK, Pandey M, Gupta S. Chamomile, a novel and selective COX-2 inhibitor with anti-inflammatory activity. *Life Sci.* 2009 Nov 4;85(19-20):663-9. PMID: 19788894. "Our data suggest that chamomile works by a mechanism of action similar to that attributed to non-steroidal anti-inflammatory drugs."

Wustrow TP et al. Alternative versus conventional treatment strategy in uncomplicated acute otitis media in children: a prospective, open, controlled, parallel-group comparison. *Int J Clin Pharmacol Ther.* 2004 Feb;42(2):110-9. PMID 15180172. Treatment with Otovowen (a propietary natural medicine including homeopathics and chamomile tincture) when compared to antibiotics resulted in fewer analgesics, and fewer days to recovery, fewer days missed from school, and was better tolerated by the children.

Chia seeds

Mohdi Ali N, Yeap KS et al. The promising future of chia, *Salvia hispanica* L. *J Biomed Biotechnol.* 2012; 171956. PMID: 23251075. "This paper covers the up-to-date research on the identified active ingredients, methods for oil extraction, and in vivo and human trials on the health benefit of chia seed" including (in human studies) cardioprotective, weight loss, reduction of triglycerides and blood glucose levels.

Chicken soup

Rennard BO, Ertl RF, et al. Chicken soup inhibits neutrophil chemotaxis in vitro. *Chest* 2000 Oct;118(4):1150-7. PMID: 11035691. "The present study ... suggests that chicken soup may contain a number of substances with beneficial medicinal activity. A mild anti-inflammatory effect could be one mechanism by which the soup could result in the mitigation of symptomatic upper respiratory tract infections."

Chocolate *(research on theobromine, the active ingredient in chocolate; theobromine is an isomer of theophylline; both are xanthine derivatives)*

Mokry J, Nosalova G, Mokra D. Influence of xanthine derivatives on cough and airway reactivity in guinea pigs. *J Physiol Pharmacol* 2009 Nov;60 Suppl;5:87-91. PMID: 20134046. "Both [theophylline and theobromine] effectively suppressed cough and made significant bronchodilation [with] more pronounced effects in ovalbumin-sensitized animals (with airway hyperresponsiveness)."

Usmani OS, Belvisi MG et al. Theobromine inhibits sensory nerve activation and cough. *FASEB J.* 2005 Feb;19(2):231-3. PMID: 15548587. "In a randomized, double-blind, placebo-controlled study in man, theobromine suppresses capsaicin-induced cough with no adverse effects. ... Theobromine directly inhibits capsaicin-induced sensory nerve depolarization of guinea-pig and human vagus nerve suggestive of an inhibitory effect on afferent nerve activation."

Cinnamon

Hayashi K, Imanishi N et al. Inhibitory effect of cinnamaldehyde, derived from *Cinnamomi* cortex, on the growth of influenza A/PR/8 virus in vitro and in vivo.

Antiviral Res. 2007 Apr;74(1):1-8. PMID: 17303260. "CA [one of the principal constituents of cinnamon essential oil] inhibited the growth [of influenza A/PR/I virus in vitro] in a dose-dependent manner (20-200 microM), and, at 200 microM, the virus yield was reduced to an undetectable level."

Ibrahim YK, Ogunmodede MS. Growth and survival of *Pseudomonas aeruginosa* in some aromatic waters. *Pharm Acta Helv.* 1991;66(9-10):286-8. PMID: 1758905. "Results showed that cinnamon water possesses profound and useful preservative activity against *Ps. aeruginosa.*"

Zhuang M, Jiang H et al. Procyanidins and butanol extract of *Cinnamomi Cortex* [cinnamon bark] inhibit SARS-CoV infection. *Antiviral Res.* 2009 Apr;82(1):73-81. Epub 2009 Feb 11. PMID: 19428598. "We found that the butanol fraction of *Cinnamomi Cortex* (CC/Fr.2) showed moderate inhibitory activity in wild-type severe acute respiratory syndrome coronavirus (wtSARS-CoV) and HIV/SARS-CoV S pseudovirus infections."

Cloves

Pawar VC, Thaker VS. In vitro efficacy of 75 essential oils against *Aspergillus niger.* Mycoses. 2006 Jul;49(4):316-23. PMID: 16784447. "[Four forms of cinnamon plus clove] were the top five essential oils which demonstrated marked inhibitory effect against hyphal growth and spore formation of A. niger."

Saini A, Sharma S, Chhibber S. Induction of resistance to respiratory tract infection with *Klebsiella pneumoniae* in mice fed on a diet supplemented with tulsi *(Ocimum sanctum)* and clove *(Syzgium aromaticum)* oils. *J Microbiol Immunol Infect.* 2009 Apr;42(2):107-13. PMID: 19597641. "The results showed that there was a significant decrease in bacterial colonization after short-term feeding with clove oil compared with the controls (p<0.05)."

Coffee

Horiuchi Y, Toda M et al. Protective activity of tea and catechins against *Bordetella pertussis. Kansenshogaku Zasshi.* 1992 May;66(5):599-605. PMID: 1402092. "Green tea, black tea and coffee showed marked bactericidal activity [against *Bordetella pertussis*] at their concentrations in beverages."

Nettleton JA, Follis JL, Schabath MB. Coffee intake, smoking, and pulmonary function in the Atherosclerosis Risk in Communities Study. *Am J Epidemiol.* 2009 Jun 15;169(12):1445-53. PMID: 19372215. "Pulmonary function values increased across increasing categories of coffee consumption in never and former smokers but not in current smokers."

Raeessi MA, Aslani J et al. Honey plus coffee versus systemic steroid in the treatment of persistent post-infectious cough: a randomised controlled trial. *Primary Care Respiratory J,* 2013 Sept;22(3) 325-30. PMID: 23966217. "Honey plus coffee was found to be the most effective treatment modality for PPC [compared to prednisolone or guaifenesin]."

Colloidal silver

Abdel Rahim KA, Ali Mohamed AM. Bactericidal and antibiotic synergistic effect of nanosilver against methicillin-resistant Staphylococcus aureus. *Jundishapur J Micro-*

biol. 2015 Nov 21;8(11):e25867. PMID: 26862383. "Methicillin-Resistant Staphylococcus aureus cells were treated with 50, 100 and 200 μg/mL of Ag-NPs and inhibited bacterial growth so that after four hours, almost all treated MRSA cells were dead. All combinations showed effectiveness against MRSA. It was observed that MRSA did not show inhibition zones with ampicillin alone."

Rai M, Yadav A, Gade A. Silver nanoparticles as a new generation of antimicrobials. *Biotechnol Adv.* 2009 Jan-Feb;27(1):76-83. PMID: 18854209. "Metallic silver in the form of silver nanoparticles has made a remarkable comeback as a potential antimicrobial agent. The use of silver nanoparticles is also important, as several pathogenic bacteria have developed resistance against various antibiotics."

Shahverdi AR, Fakhimi A et al. Synthesis and effect of silver nanoparticles on the antibacterial activity of different antibiotics against *Staphylococcus aureus* and *E. coli.* *Nanomedicine.* 2007 Jun;3(2):168-71. PMID: 17468052. "The antibacterial activities of penicillin G, amoxicillin, erythromycin, clindamycin, and vancomycin were increased in the presence of Ag-NPs [silver nanoparticles] against both test strains. The highest enhancing effects were observed for vancomycin, amoxicillin, and penicillin G against *S. aureus.* "

CoQ10 (Coenzyme Q10)

Papas KA, Sontag MK et al. A pilot study on the safety and efficacy of a novel antioxidant rich formulation in patients with cystic fibrosis. *J Cyst Fibros.* 2008 Jan; 7(1):60-7. PMID: 17569601. "The novel CF-1 formulation safely and effectively increased plasma levels of important fat-soluble nutrients and antioxidants. In addition, improvements in antioxidant plasma levels were associated with reductions in airway inflammation in CF patients."

Schmelzer C, Lindner I et al. Functions of coenzyme Q10 in inflammation and gene expression. *Biofactors.* 2008;32(1-4):179-83. PMID: 19096114. "The in silico analysis as well as the cell culture experiments suggested that CoQ10 exerts anti-inflammatory properties via NFkappaB1-dependent gene expression."

Schmelzer C, Lorenz G et al. In vitro effects of the reduced form of coenzyme Q(10) on secretion levels of TNF-alpha and chemokines in response to LPS in the human monocytic cell line THP-1. *J Clin Biochem Nutr.* 2009 Jan;44(1):62-6. PMID: 19177190 "Our results indicate anti-inflammatory effects of the reduced form of CoQ(10) on various proinflammatory cytokines and chemokines in vitro."

Cordyceps

Lin XX, Xie QM et al. Effects of fermented Cordyceps powder on pulmonary function in sensitized guinea pigs and airway inflammation in sensitized rats. *Zhongguo Zhong Yao Za Zhi.* 2001 Sep;26(9):622-5. PMID: 12776432. "Cordyceps … significantly inhibited bronchial challenge of ovalbumin-induced change of RL and Cdyn (P < 0.05) and inhibited antigen-induced increase of eosinophils in the BALF of rats (P < 0.05). … Cordyceps could be applied for the prevention and cure of asthma."

Ohta Y, Lee JB et al. In vivo anti-influenza virus activity of an immunomodulatory acidic polysaccharide [APS] isolated from *Cordyceps militaris* grown on germinated soybeans. *J Agric Food Chem.* 2007 Dec 12;55(25):10194-9. PMID: 17988090. "APS might have beneficial therapeutic effects on influenza A virus infection at least in part by modulation of the immune function of macrophages."

Wang NQ, Jiang LD et al. Effect of dongchong xiacao [cordyceps] capsule on airway inflammation of asthmatic patients. *Zhongguo Zhong Yao Za Zhi.* 2007 Aug;32(15):1566-8. PMID: 17972591. "[Corcyceps] can reduce the serum markers of airway inflammation, which suggests this therapy bears the anti-inflammation effects probably through regulating the balance of TH1/TH2, inhibiting the activity of adherence molecule and reducing IgE production. It may also have the effect of reversing airway remodeling, which needs further research to determine."

Curcumin

Kuptniratsaikul V, Dajpratham P et al. Efficacy and safety of *Curcuma domestica* extracts compared with ibuprofen in patients with knee osteoarthritis: a multicenter study. *Clin Interv Aging.* 2014 Mar 20;9:451-8. PMID: 24672232. "[Curcumin] extracts are as effective as ibuprofen for the treatment of knee osteoarthritis. The side effect profile was similar but with fewer gastrointestinal AE reports in the [curcumin] group."

Chandran B, Goel A. A randomized, pilot study to assess the efficacy and safety of curcumin in patients with active rheumatoid arthritis. *Phytother Res.* 2012 Nov;26(11):1719-25. PMID: 22407780. "The curcumin group showed the highest percentage of improvement in overall DAS and ACR scores (ACR 20, 50 and 70) and these scores were significantly better than the patients in the diclofenac sodium group. More importantly, curcumin treatment was found to be safe and did not relate with any adverse events."

Echinacea

Cohen HA, Varsano I et al. Effectiveness of an herbal preparation containing echinacea, propolis, and vitamin C in preventing respiratory tract infections in children: a randomized, double-blind, placebo-controlled, multicenter study. *Arch Pediatr Adolesc Med.* 2004 Mar;158(3):217-21. PMID: 14993078. "Significant ... reductions of illnesses were seen in the [herbal] group in the number of illness episodes; number of episodes per child; and number of days with fever per child. The total number of illness days and duration of individual episodes were also significantly lower in the [herbal] group. Adverse drug reactions were rare, mild, and transient."

Melchart D, Linde K et al. Echinacea for preventing and treating the common cold. *Cochrane Database Syst Rev.* 2000(2):CD000530. PMID: 10796553. "Sixteen trials (eight prevention trials, and eight trials on treatment of upper respiratory tract infections) with a total of 3396 participants were included. ...The majority of the available studies report positive results."

Schapowal A, Berger D et al. Echinacea/sage or chlorhexidine/lidocaine for treating acute sore throats: a randomized double-blind trial. *Eur J Med Res.* 2009 Sep 1;14(9):406-12. PMID: 19748859. "The echinacea/sage treatment exhibited similar efficacy to the chlorhexidine/lidocaine treatment in reducing sore throat symptoms during the first 3 days (P(x<Y) = .5083). Response rates after 3 days were 63.8% in

the echinacea/sage group and 57.8% in the chlorhexidine/lidocaine group."

Shah SA, Sander S et al. Evaluation of echinacea for the prevention and treatment of the common cold: a meta-analysis. *Lancet Infect Dis.* 2007 Jul;7(7):473-80. PMID: 17597571. "Echinacea decreased the odds of developing the common cold by 58% (OR 0.42; 95% CI 0.25-0.71; Q statistic p<0.001) and the duration of a cold by 1.4 days (WMD -1.44, -2.24 to -0.64; p=0.01)." At least two of the 14 studies reviewed included children.

Elderberry

Roschek B, Fink RC et al. Elderberry flavonoids bind to and prevent H1N1 infection in vitro. *Phytochemistry.* 2009 Jul;70(10):1255-61. PMID: 19682714. "The H1N1 inhibition activities of the elderberry flavonoids compare favorably to the known anti-influenza activities of Oseltamivir (0.32 microM) and Amantadine (27 microM)."

Wustrow TP et al. Alternative versus conventional treatment strategy in uncomplicated acute otitis media in children: a prospective, open, controlled-parallel group comparison. *Int J Clin Pharmacol Ther.* 2004 Feb;42(2):110-9. PMID 15180172. Treatment with Otovowen (a proprietary natural medicine including homeopathics and elderberry) when compared to antibiotics resulted in fewer analgesics, fewer days to recovery, fewer days missed from school, and was better tolerated by the children.

Zakay-Rones Z, Thom E et al. Randomized study of the efficacy and safety of oral elderberry extract in the treatment of influenza A and B virus infections. *J Int Med Res.* 2004 Mar-Apr;32(2):132-40. PMID: 15080016. "Symptoms were relieved on average 4 days earlier and use of rescue medication was significantly less in those receiving elderberry extract compared with placebo."

Zakay-Rones Z, Varsano N et al. Inhibition of several strains of influenza virus in vitro and reduction of symptoms by an elderberry extract (Sambucus nigra L.) during an outbreak of influenza B Panama. *J Altern Complement Med.* 1995 Winter;1(4):361-9. PMID: 9395631. "A complete cure was achieved within 2 to 3 days in nearly 90% of the Sambucol-treated group and within at least 6 days in the placebo group (p < 0.001)."

Enzymes

Lanchava N, Nemsadze K et al. Wobenzym in treatment of recurrent obstructive bronchitis in children. *Georgian Med News.* 2005 Oct;(127):50-3. PMID: 16308444. "Analysis of the data, obtained after treatment, demonstrated decrease of the Daily Symptom Score and an increase of Symptom Free Days, as well as an improvement in spirometric indices (FVC, FEV, PEF)."

Essential fatty acids, see Fish Oil

Eucalyptus

Ben-Arye E, Dudai N et al. Treatment of upper respiratory tract infections in primary care: a randomized study using aromatic herbs. *Evid Based Complement Alternat Med.* 2011;2011:690346. PMID: 21052500. "In conclusion, spray application of [a blend of eucalyptus, peppermint, oregano and rosemary oils] ... brings about significant and immediate improvement in symptoms of upper respiratory ailment."

Salari MH, Amine G et al. Antibacterial effects of *Eucalyptus globulus* leaf extract on pathogenic bacteria isolated from specimens of patients with respiratory tract disorders. *Clin Microbiol Infect.* 2006 Feb;12(2):194-6. PMID: 16441463. "The anti-bacterial activity of *Eucalyptus globulus* leaf extract was determined for 56 isolates of *Staphylococcus aureus,* 25 isolates of *Streptococcus pyogenes,* 12 isolates of *Streptococcus pneumoniae* and seven isolates of *Haemophilus influenzae* obtained from 200 clinical specimens of patients with respiratory tract disorders. MIC50s for these species were 64, 32, 16 and 16 mg/L, respectively; MIC90s were 128, 64, 32 and 32 mg/L, respectively; and MBCs were 512, 128, 64 and 64 mg/L, respectively."

Feverfew

Diener HC, Pfaffenrath V et al. Efficacy and safety of 6.25 mg t.i.d. feverfew CO_2-extract (MIG-99) in migraine prevention--a randomized, double-blind, multi-centre, placebo-controlled study. *Cephalalgia.* 2005 Nov;25(11):1031-41. PMID: 16232154. "The migraine frequency decreased from 4.76 by 1.9 attacks per month in the MIG-99 group and by 1.3 attacks in the placebo group (P = 0.0456) ... odds ratio of 3.4 in favour of MIG-99 (P = 0.0049). Adverse events possibly related to study medication were 9/107 (8.4%) with MIG-99 and 11/108 (10.2%) with placebo (P = 0.654)."

Shrivastava R, Pechadre JC, John GW. *Tanacetum parthenium* [feverfew] and *Salix alba* [white willow] (Mig-RL) combination in migraine prophylaxis: a prospective, open-label study. *Clin Drug Investig.* 2006;26(5):287-96. Shrivastava R, Pechadre JC, John GW. Tanacetum parthenium [feverfew] and Salix alba [white willow] (Mig-RL) combination in migraine prophylaxis: a prospective, open-label study. "The remarkable efficacy of Mig-RL in not only reducing the frequency of migraine attacks but also their pain intensity and duration in this trial warrants further investigation."

Fish oil/essential fatty acids

Biltagi MA, Baset AA et al. Omega-3 fatty acids, vitamin C and Zn supplementation in asthmatic children: a randomized self-controlled study. *Acta Paediatr.* 2009 Apr;98(4):737-42. PMID: 19154523. "There was a significant improvement of C-ACT, pulmonary function tests and sputum inflammatory markers with diet supplementation with omega-3 fatty acids, vitamin C and Zn (p < 0.001*)."

Calder PC. N-3 polyunsaturated fatty acids and inflammation: from molecular biology to the clinic. *Lipids.* 2003 Apr;38(4):343-52. PMID: 12848278 "Clinical studies have reported that oral fish oil supplementation has beneficial effects in rheumatoid arthritis and among some asthmatics, supporting the idea that the n-3 FA in fish oil are anti-inflammatory."

Nagakura T, Matsuda S et al. Dietary supplementation with fish oil rich in omega-3 polyunsaturated fatty acids in children with bronchial asthma. *Eur Respir J.* 2000 Nov;16(5):861-5. PMID: 11153584. "Asthma symptom scores decreased and responsiveness to acetylcholine decreased in the fish oil group but not in the control group."

Tecklenburg-Lund S, Mickleborough TD et al. Randomized controlled trial of fish oil and montelukast and their combination on airway inflammation and hyperpnea-induced bronchoconstriction. *PLoS One.* 2010 Oct 18;5(10):e13487. PMID: 20976161. "Fish oil and montelukast [Singulair] are both effective in attenuating airway inflammation and HIB [hyperpnea-induced bronchoconstriction] … Fish oil supplementation should be considered as an alternative treatment for EIB [exercise-induced bronchoconstriction].

Fritillary

Li SY, Li JS et al. Effects of comprehensive therapy based on traditional Chinese medicine patterns in stable chronic obstructive pulmonary disease: a four-center, open-label, randomized, controlled study. *BMC Complement Altern Med.* 2012 Oct 29;12:197. PMID: 23107470. Fritillary was a component of one of the three Traditional Chinese Medicine [TCM] blends used according to TCM diagnosis. "Both the primary outcomes of this study [acute exacerbation of COPD and lung function measured by FEV_1 and dyspnea score] were significantly improved with TCM."

Garlic

Arzanlou M, Bohlooli S et al. Allicin from garlic neutralizes the hemolytic activity of intra- and extra-cellular pneumolysin O in vitro. *Toxicon.* 2011 Mar 15;57(4):540-5. PMID: 21184771 "Exposure of intact cells to allicin (1.8 μM) completely inhibited haemolytic activity of pneumolysin inside bacterial cells. The inhibitory effect of the allicin was restored by addition of reducing agent DTT at 5 mM, proposing that allicin likely inhibits the pneumolysin by binding to cysteinyl residue in the binding site. The MIC value of allicin was determined to be 512 μg/mL (3.15 μM/mL). These results indicate that PLY is a novel target for allicin and may provide a new line of investigation on pneumococcal diseases in the future."

Hannan A, Ikram Ullah M et al. Anti-mycobacterial activity of garlic *(Allium sativum)* against multi-drug resistant and non-multi-drug resistant mycobacterium tuberculosis. *Pak J Pharm Sci.* 2011 Jan;24(1):81-5. PMID: 21190924. "Minimum inhibitory concentration (MIC) of garlic extract ranged from 1 to 3 mg/ml, showing inhibitory effects of garlic against both non-MDR and MDR *M. tuberculosis* isolates."

Karuppia P, Rajaram S. Antibacterial effect of *Allium sativum* cloves and *Zingiber officinale* rhizomes against multiple-drug resistant clinical pathogens. *Asian Pac J Trop Biomed.* 2012 Aug;2(8):597-601. PMID: 23569978. "The highest inhibition zone was observed with garlic (19.45 mm) against *Pseudomonas aeruginosa.*"

Ginger

Chang JS, Wang KC et al. Fresh ginger *(Zingiber officinale)* has anti-viral activity against human respiratory syncytial virus in human respiratory tract cell lines. *J Ethnopharmacol.* 2013 Jan 9;145(1):146-51. PMID: 23123794. "Fresh ginger dose-dependently inhibited viral attachment (p<0.0001) and internalization (p<0.0001). … [It] is effective against HRSV-induced plaque formation on airway epithelium by blocking viral attachment and internalization."

Denyer CV, Jackson P et al. Isolation of antirhinoviral sesquiterpenes from ginger *(Zingiber officinale). J Nat Prod.* 1994 May;57(5):658-62. PMID: 8064299. "The most active of these [ginger sesquiterpenes] was beta-sesquiphellandrene [2] with an IC50 of 0.44 microM vs. rhinovirus IB in vitro."

Shariatpanahi ZV, Taleban FA et al. Ginger extract reduces delayed gastric emptying and nosocomial pneumonia in adult respiratory distress syndrome patients hospitalized in an intensive care unit. *J Crit Care.* 2010 Dec;25(4):647-50. PMID: 20149584. "There was a trend toward a decrease in pneumonia in the ginger group (P = .07)....Gastric feed supplementation with ginger extract might reduce delayed gastric emptying and help reduce the incidence of ventilator-associated pneumonia in ARDS."

Ginseng *see* **American ginseng**

Goldenseal

Cech NB, Junio HA. Quorum quenching and antimicrobial activity of golden-seal (Hydrastis canadensis) against methicillin-resistant Staphylococcus aureus (MRSA). *Planta Med.* 2012 Sep;78(14):1556-61. PMID: 22814821. "The H. canaden-sis leaf extract (but not the isolated alkaloids berberine, hydrastine, and canadine) demonstrated quorum quenching activity against several clinically relevant MRSA isolates (USA300 strains). Our data suggest that this occurs by attenuation of sig-nal transduction through the AgrCA two-component system. Consistent with this observation, the extract inhibited toxin production by MRSA and prevented dam-age by MRSA to keratinocyte cells in vitro."

Green tea *see* **Tea, green or black**

Grindelia (herbal; see Appendix E for research on its homeopathic use)

Brinker F. Herbs and drugs in the treatment of respiratory allergies. *British Naturo-pathic Journal* 17(3):50-53, 2000. Various species of Grindelia "contain flavonoids quercitin and luteolin and are used as expectorants and mild antispasmodics that inhibit histamine release."

Homeopathic remedies, see Appendix E

Honey

Henriques AF, Jenkins RE et al. The effect of manuka honey on the structure of *Pseu-domonas aeruginosa. Eur J Clin Microbiol Infect Dis.* 2011 Feb ;30(2):167-71. PMID: 20936493 "The MIC and MBC values of manuka honey against *P. aeruginosa* were 9.5% (w/v) and 12% (w/v) respectively; a time-kill curve demonstrated a bactericidal rather than a bacteriostatic effect, with a 5 log reduction estimated within 257 min. … manuka honey has the potential to be an effective inhibitor of *P. aeruginosa.*"

Paul IM, Beiler J et al. Effect of honey, dextromethorphan, and no treatment on noc-turnal cough and sleep quality for coughing children and their parents. *Arch Pedi-atr Adolesc Med.* 2007 Dec ;161(12):1140-6. PMID: 18056558. "In a comparison of [buckwheat] honey, DM [dextromethorphan], and no treatment, parents rated honey most favorably for symptomatic relief of their child's nocturnal cough and sleep difficulty due to upper respiratory tract infection."

Raeessi MA, Aslani J et al. Honey plus coffee versus systemic steroid in the treatment of persistent post-infectious cough: a randomised controlled trial. *Primary Care Respiratory Journal,* 2013 Sept;22(3):325-30. PMID: 23966217. "The mean (+/- SD) cough scores pre- and post-treatmexent were: HC group 2.9 (0.3) pre-treatment and 0.2 (0.5) post-treatment (p<0.001); steroid ('S') group 3.0 (0.0) pre-treatment and 2.4 (0.6) post-treatment (p<0.05); control ('C') group 2.8 (0.4) pre-treatment and 2.7 (0.5) post-treatment (p>0.05). … Honey plus coffee was found to be the most effective treatment modality for PPC."

Watanabe K, Rahmasari R et al. Anti-influenza viral effects of honey in vitro: potent high activity of manuka honey. *Arch Med Res.* 2014 Jul;45(5):359-65. PMID: 24880005. "Manuka honey efficiently inhibited influenza virus replication. ... In the presence of manuka honey, the IC50 of zanamir or oseltamivir was reduced to nearly 1/1000th of their single use."

Horseradish

Esanu V, Prahoveanu E. The effect of an aqueous horse-radish extract, applied as such or in association with caffeine, on experimental influenza in mice. *Virologie.* 1985 Apr-Jun;36(2):95-8. PMID: 4036004. "The antiviral effect of the extract [on influenza virus A/PR8/34 (H1N1)]—also demonstrated in vitro—-was reflected by a significant decrease in the hemagglutination titers recorded in mouse lung homogenates and by a slight increase in the mean survival time of treated mice versus untreated controls."

Yano Y, Satomi M, Oikawa H. Antimicrobial effect of spices and herbs on *Vibrio parahaemolyticus. Int J Food Microbiol.* 2006 Aug 15;111(1):6-11. PMID: 16797760. "Basil, clove, garlic, horseradish, marjoram, oregano, rosemary, and thyme exhibited antibacterial activities [against *Vibrio parahaemolyticus*] at incubation of 30° C."

Ivy

Kemmerich B, Eberhardt R, Stammer H. Efficacy and tolerability of a fluid extract combination of thyme herb and ivy leaves and matched placebo in adults suffering from acute bronchitis with productive cough. A prospective, double-blind, placebo-controlled clinical trial. *Arzneimittelforschung.* 2006;56(9):652-60. PMID 17063641. "The symptoms of acute bronchitis (BSS) improved rapidly in both groups, but regression of symptoms was faster and the responder rates (p<0.0001) compared to placebo were higher at Visit 2 (83.0% vs 53.9%) and Visit 3 (96.2% vs. 74.7%) under the treatment of thyme-ivy combination."

Lavender

Roller S, Ernest N, Buckle J. The antimicrobial activity of high-necrodane and other lavender oils on methicillin-sensitive and -resistant Staphylococcus aureus (MSSA and MRSA). *J Altern Complement Med.* 2009 Mar;15(3):275-9. PMID: 19249919. "All four lavender oils inhibited growth of both MSSA and MRSA by direct contact but not in the vapor phase. Inhibition zones ranged from 8 to 30 mm in diameter ... demonstrating a dose response."

Lemon

de Castillo MC, de Allori CG et al. Bactericidal activity of lemon juice and lemon derivatives against *Vibrio cholerae. Biol Pharm Bull.* 2000 Oct;23(10):1235-8. PMID: 11041258. "Concentrated lemon juice and essential oils inhibited *V. cholerae* completely at all studied dilutions and exposure times. ... Freshly squeezed lemon juice, diluted to 10(-2), showed complete inhibition of *V. cholerae* at a concentration of 10(8) CFU ml(-1) after 5 min of exposure time ... It can be concluded that lemon, a natural product which is easily obtained, acts as a biocide against *V. cholerae,* and is, therefore, an efficient decontaminant, harmless to humans."

Grassmann J, Schneider D et al. Antioxidative effects of lemon oil and its components on copper induced oxidation of low density lipoprotein. *Arzneimittelforschung.* 2001 Oct;51(10):799-805. PMID: 11715632 "To follow the kinetics of copper induced LDL-oxidation, formation of conjugated dienes as well as loss of tryptophan fluorescence were measured. ... Lemon oil and one of its components, gamma-terpinene, are efficiently slowing down the oxidation of LDL."

Licorice

Cinatl J, Morgenstern B, et al. Glycyrrhizin, an active component of liquorice roots, and replication of SARS-associated coronavirus. *Lancet* 2003 Jun 14;361(9374):2045-6. PMID: 12814717. "We assessed the antiviral potential of ribavirin, 6-azauridine, pyrazofurin, mycophenolic acid, and glycyrrhizin against two clinical isolates of coronavirus (FFM-1 and FFM-2) from patients with SARS admitted to the clinical centre of Frankfurt University, Germany. Of all the compounds, glycyrrhizin was the most active in inhibiting replication of the SARS-associated virus."

Karimov MM. Use of extracts of *Glycerrhiza glabra* [licorice] in the correction of some indices of local nonspecific defense in patients with protracted pulmonary pneumonia. *Lik Sprava.* 2001 Sep-Dec;(5-6):123-5. PMID: 11881346. "[Licorice extract was]superior to T-activin in diminishing neutrophilic granulocytes count and increasing the BALF content of macrophages, lysozyme, s IgA; it proved to be endowed with an antiphospholipase activity, which [indicate effectiveness in] patients presenting with protracted pneumonia."

Long DR, Mead J et al. 18beta-Glycyrrhetinic acid inhibits MRSA survival and attenuates virulence gene expression. *Antimicrob Agents Chemother.* 2013 Jan;57(1):241-7. PMID: 23114775. "At high concentrations [licorice extract] is bactericidal to MRSA and at sublethal doses reduces virulence gene expression in *S. aureus* both in vitro and in vivo."

Xie Y-C, Dong X-W et al. Inhibitory effects of flavonoids extracted from licorice on lipopolysaccharide-induced acute pulmonary inflammation in mice. *Int Immunopharmacol.* 2009 Feb;9(2):194-200. PMID: 19071231. "We suggest that licorice flavonoids effectively attenuate LPS-induced pulmonary inflammation through inhibition of inflammatory cells infiltration and inflammatory mediator release which subsequently reduces neutrophil recruitment into lung and neutrophil-mediated oxidative injury."

Lime

Rahman S, Parvez AK et al. Antibacterial activity of natural spices on multiple drug resistant Escherichia coli isolated from drinking water, Bangladesh. *Ann Clin Microbiol Antimicrob.* 2011 Mar 15;10:10. PMID: 21406097 "All the bacterial isolates were susceptible to undiluted lime-juice. The highest inhibition zone was observed with lime (11 mm). [Lime] could be used for prevention of diarrheal diseases."

Loquat

Ge JF, Wang TY et al. Anti-inflammatory effect of triterpenoic acids of *Eriobotrya japonica* (Thunb.) Lindl. leaf on rat model of chronic bronchitis. *Am J Chin Med.* 2009;37(2):309-21. PMID: 19507274. "As compared to the normal and sham groups, the total number of leukocyte, the differential counts of neutrophils and alveolar macrophage (AM) in BALF, the levels of TNF-alpha and IL-8 in the super-

Menthol

Eccles, R. Menthol: from folklore to pharmacology. *International Pharmacy Journal,* Vol. 6, 1995, pp. 23-24. "One study showed that Vicks VapoRub [a blend of menthol, camphor and eucalyptus] worked better than pseudoephedrine at relieving nasal congestion."

Hamoud R, Sporer F et al. Antimicrobial activity of a traditionally used complex essential oil distillate (Olbas(*) Tropfen) in comparison to its individual essential oil ingredients. *Phytomedicine.* 2012 Aug 15;19(11):969-76. PMID: 22739414. "[Olbas's] antimicrobial activity was comparable to that of peppermint oil which was the most potent one of all individual essential oils tested. Based on its wide antimicrobial properties Olbas can be a useful agent for the treatment of uncomplicated infections of skin and respiratory tract."

Klyachkina IL. [The new possibility for the treatment of acute cough] *Vestn Otorinolaringol.* 2015;80(5):85-90. PMID: 26525480 "The volatile metabolites of ambroxol [including] menthol and cineol exert the mucolytic, antiseptic, and antibacterial actions, after they reach the trachea and bronchi. Irrigation of the receptors present in the inflamed mucous membrane of the larynx, pharynx, and nasal cavity, with these volatile substances produces an immediate cough-suppressive effect [and] the excretion of viscous and difficult-of-discharge bronchial mucus."

N-acetylcysteine (NAC)

Rochat T, Lacroix JS, Jornot L. N-acetylcysteine inhibits Na+ absorption across human nasal epithelial cells. *J Cell Physiol* 2004 Oct;201(1)106-16. PMID 15281093. "N-acetylcysteine (NAC) is a widely used mucolytic drug in patients with a variety of respiratory disorders. The mechanism of action is based on rupture of the disulfide bridges of the high molecular glycoproteins present in the mucus, resulting in smaller subunits of the glycoproteins and reduced viscosity of the mucus [causing an] increase in the fluidity of the airway mucus."

Oil of oregano

Dahiya P, Purkayastha S. Phytochemical screening and antimicrobial activity of some medicinal plants against multi-drug resistant bacteria from clinical isolates. *Indian J Pharm Sci.* 2012 Sep;74(5):443-50. PMID: 23716873 "Methanol and ethanol extracts from tulsi, oregano, rosemary, lemongrass, aloe vera and thyme presented antimicrobial activity to S. aureus MRSA. Previous reports also revealed the antibacterial efficacy of the investigated plant extracts and essential oils against S. aureus MRSA."

Eng W, Norman R. Development of an oregano-based ointment with anti-microbial activity including activity against methicillin-resistant Staphlococcus aureus. *J Drugs Dermatol.* 2010 Apr;9(4):377-80. PMID: 20514796. "Disk diffusion studies showed that oregano was found to be bacteriostatic for Staphylococcus aureus (S. aureus) and methicillin-resistant S. aureus, (MRSA) but bacteriocidal for seven other microorganisms."

Preuss HG1, Echard B et al. Minimum inhibitory concentrations of herbal essential oils and monolaurin for gram-positive and gram-negative bacteria. *Mol Cell Biochem.*

2005 Apr;272(1-2):29-34. PMID: 16010969. "Origanum proved cidal to all tested organisms [*Staphylococcus aureus, Bacillus anthracis* Sterne, *Escherichia coli, Klebsiella pneumoniae, Helicobacter pylori,* and *Mycobacterium terrae*] with the exception of *B. anthracis* Sterne in which it was static. ... Because of their longstanding safety record, origanum and/or monolaurin, alone or combined with antibiotics, might prove useful in the prevention and treatment of severe bacterial infections, especially those that are difficult to treat and/or are antibiotic resistant."

Olive leaf extract

Pereira AP, Ferreira IC et al. Phenolic compounds and antimicrobial activity of olive (*Olea europaea* L. Cv. Cobrançosa) leaves. *Molecules.* 2007 May 26;12(5):1153-62. PMID: 17873849. "We report ... their in vitro activity against ... gram positive (Bacillus cereus, B. subtilis and Staphylococcus aureus), gram negative bacteria (Pseudomonas aeruginosa, Escherichia coli and Klebsiella pneumoniae) and fungi (Candida albicans and Cryptococcus neoformans)....At low concentrations olive leaves extracts showed an unusual combined antibacterial and antifungal action, which suggest their great potential as nutraceuticals, particularly as a source of phenolic compounds."

Pelargonium

Matthys H, Funk P. EPs 7630 improves acute bronchitic symptoms and shortens time to remission. Results of a randomised, double-blind, placebo-controlled, multi-centre trial. *Planta Med.* 2008 May;74(6):686-92. PMID: 18449849. "As compared with placebo, a marked improvement has been shown for EPs 7630 [Pelargonium standardized extract] for all disease symptoms (cough, sputum, rales, dyspnoe, pain on coughing, hoarseness, headache, fatigue, fever, limb pain) categorised in severity classes by the patient. Especially strong antitussive and 'anti-fatigue' effects with an early onset during treatment were observed."

Matthys H, Heger M. Treatment of acute bronchitis with a liquid herbal drug preparation from *Pelargonium sidoides* (EPs 7630): a randomized, double-blind, placebo-controlled, multicentre study. *Curr Med Res Opin.* 2007 Feb;23(2):323-31. PMID: 17288687 "EPs 7630-solution is a well tolerated and effective treatment for acute bronchitis in adults outside the very restricted indication for an antibiotic therapy."

Michaelis M, Doerr WH, Cinatl J Jr. Investigation of the influence of EPs® 7630, a herbal drug preparation from *Pelargonium sidoides*, on replication of a broad panel of respiratory viruses. *Phytomedicine.* 2011 Mar 15;18(5):384-6. PMID: 21036571. "Antiviral effects may contribute to the beneficial effects exerted by EPs(®) 7630 in acute bronchitis patients."

Peppermint see Menthol (its active ingredient, found in peppermint and other mints)
Pine

Vigo E, Cepeda A et al. In-vitro anti-inflammatory activity of *Pinus sylvestris* and *Plantago lanceolata* extracts: effect on inducible NOS, COX-1, COX-2 and their products in J774A.1 murine macrophages. *J Pharm Pharmacol.* 2005 Mar;57(3):383-91. PMID: 15807995. "The anti-inflammatory properties of *Pinus sylvestris* and *Plantago lanceolata* [plantain] extracts may reflect decreased NO [nitric oxide] production, possibly due to inhibitory effects on iNOS gene expression or to NO-scavenging activity."

Platycodon (oleanane triterpenes are the active ingredients as well as in olive oil and ginseng)

Liu J. Pharmacology of oleanolic acid and ursolic acid. *J Ethnopharmacol.* 1995 Dec 1;49(2):57-68. PMID: 8847885. "Oleanolic acid and ursolic acid have been long-recognized to have antiinflammatory and antihyperlipidemic properties in laboratory animals ...Recently, both compounds have been noted for their antitumor-promotion effects ... [They] are relatively non-toxic."

Probiotics

Agüero G, Villena J et al. Beneficial immunomodulatory activity of *Lactobacillus casei* in malnourished mice pneumonia: effect on inflammation and coagulation. *Nutrition.* 2006 Jul-Aug;22(7-8):810-9. PMID: 16815495. "Repletion with supplemental *L. casei* accelerated recovery of the defense mechanisms against pneumococci by inducing different cytokine profiles. These cytokines would be involved in the improvement of the immune response and in the induction of a more efficient regulation of the inflammatory process, limiting the injury caused by infection."

Ivory K, Chambers SJ et al. Oral delivery of *Lactobacillus casei Shirota* modifies allergen-induced immune responses in allergic rhinitis. *Clin Exp Allergy.* 2008 Aug;38(8):1282-9. PMID: 18510694. "Changes in antigen-induced production of cytokines were observed in patients treated with probiotics. These data show that probiotic supplementation modulates immune responses in allergic rhinitis and may have the potential to alleviate the severity of symptoms."

Leyer GJ, Li S et al. Probiotic effects on cold and influenza-like symptom incidence and duration in children. *Pediatrics.* 2009 Aug;124(2):e172-9. PMID: 19651563. "Daily dietary probiotic supplementation for 6 months was a safe effective way to reduce fever, rhinorrhea, and cough incidence and duration and antibiotic prescription incidence, as well as the number of missed school days attributable to illness, for children 3 to 5 years of age."

Shepeleva IB, Zakharova NS et al. Effect of blastolysin on the development of specific immunity to whooping cough. *Zh Mikrobiol Epidemiol Immunobiol.* 1986 Jan;(1):62-5. PMID: 3705806. "The use of blastolysin, the cell-wall glycopeptide of *Lactobacillus bulgaricus,*, introduced as a stimulating agent in definite doses and following definite administration schedules, has been shown to permit achieving not only an increase in the immunogenicity of the corpuscular pertussis vaccine, but also a considerable decrease in its toxicity and histamine-sensitizing activity."

Shimizu K, Ogura H et al. Synbiotics decrease the incidence of septic complications in patients with severe SIRS [systemic inflammatory response syndrome]: a preliminary report. *Dig Dis Sci.* 2009 May;54(5):1071-8. PMID: 18726154. "The incidence of infectious complications such as enteritis, pneumonia, and bacteremia was significantly lower in the [synbiotic] group than in the [placebo control] group. Synbiotics maintain the gut flora and environment and decrease the incidence of septic complications in patients with severe SIRS."

de Vrese M, Winkler P et al. Effect of [specific probiotics] on common cold episodes:

a double blind, randomized, controlled trial. *Clin Nutr.* 2005 Aug;24(4):481-91. PMID: 16054520. "The intake of probiotic bacteria during at least 3 months significantly shortened common cold episodes by almost 2 days and reduced the severity of symptoms."

Propolis

Sforcin JM, Orsi RO, Bankova V. Effect of propolis, some isolated compounds and its source plant on antibody production. *J Ethnopharmacol.* 2005 Apr 26;98(3):301-5. PMID: 15814263. "We conclude that propolis stimulates antibody production."

Sforcin JM. Propolis and the immune system: a review. J *Ethnopharmacol.* 2007 Aug 15;113(1):1-14. PMID: 17580109. "In vitro and in vivo assays demonstrated the modulatory action of propolis on murine peritoneal macrophages, increasing their microbicidal activity. Its stimulant action on the lytic activity of natural killer cells against tumor cells, and on antibody production was demonstrated."

Reishi

Kashimoto N, Hayama M et al. Inhibitory effect of a water-soluble extract from the culture medium of *Ganoderma lucidum* (Reishi) mycelia on the development of pulmonary adenocarcinoma ... in Wistar rats. *Oncol Rep.* 2006 Dec;16(6):1181-7. PMID: 17089035. "Dietary supplementation with MAK [reishi extract] inhibits the development of lung tumors, suggesting that MAK may be a potent chemopreventive agent against lung carcinogenesis."

Sadava D, Still DW et al. Effect of *Ganoderma* [reishi] on drug-sensitive and multidrug-resistant small-cell lung carcinoma cells. *Cancer Lett.* 2009 May 18;277(2):182-9. PMID: 19188016. "Extracts of several species of *Ganoderma* are cytotoxic to both drug-sensitive and drug-resistant SCLC cells, are pro-apoptotic, induce gene expression patterns that are similar to SCLC cells treated with chemotherapeutic drugs, and can reverse resistance to chemotherapeutic drugs."

Romerillo

Onga PL, Weng BC et al. The anticancer effect of protein-extract from *Bidens alba* in human colorectal carcinoma SW480 cells via the reactive oxidative species- and glutathione depletion-dependent apoptosis. *Food and Chemical Toxicology* 2008 (May);46(5):1535-47. PMID: 18226850. "*Bidens alba* [romerillo] has been used for healing cuts, injuries, swellings, hypertension, jaundice, and diabetes in some countries.... We demonstrated ... that the protein-extract of *B. alba* could induce apoptosis that was related to the ROS production and GSH depletion in human colorectal cancer."

Rosemary

Ben-Arye E, Dudai N et al. Treatment of upper respiratory tract infections in primary care: a randomized study using aromatic herbs. *Evid Based Complement Alternat Med.* 2011;2011:690346. PMID: 21052500. "Application of five aromatic plants [including rosemary] reported in this study brings about significant and immediate improvement in symptoms of upper respiratory ailments."

Sage

Hubbert M, Sievers H et al. Efficacy and tolerability of a spray with *Salvia officinalis* in the treatment of acute pharyngitis—a randomised, double-blind, placebo-controlled study with adaptive design and interim analysis. *Eur J Med Res.* 2006 Jan 31;11(1):20-6. PMID: 16504956. "The efficacy and tolerability profile of a 15% sage spray indicated that it provides a convenient and safe treatment for patients with acute pharyngitis. A symptomatic relief occurred within the first two hours after first administration and was statistically significantly superior to placebo."

Schapowal A, Berger D et al. Echinacea/sage or chlorhexidine/lidocaine for treating acute sore throats: a randomized double-blind trial. *Eur J Med Res.* 2009 Sep 1;14(9):406-12. PMID: 19748859. "The echinacea/sage treatment exhibited similar efficacy to the chlorhexidine/lidocaine treatment in reducing sore throat symptoms during the first 3 days (P(x<Y) = .5083). Response rates [decrease of at least 50% of total symptoms] after 3 days were 63.8% in the echinacea/sage group and 57.8% in the chlorhexidine/lidocaine group."

Slippery elm

Gill RE, Hirst EL, Jones JK. Constitution of the mucilage from the bark of *Ulmus fulva* (slippery elm mucilage); the sugars formed in the hydrolysis of the methylated mucilage. *J Chem Soc.* 1946 Nov:1025-9.PMID: 20282480

Star anise

Campbell, Emily. How is Tamiflu synthesized? University of Bristol (England) website, http://www.chm.bris.ac.uk/motm/tamiflu/synthesis.htm. Tamiflu is made using shikimic acid, originally extracted from star anise, now produced by bacterial fermentation to create a larger volume at lower cost.

Park SH, Sung YY, et al. Protective activity ethanol extract of the fruits of *Illicium verum* against atherogenesis in apolipoprotein E knockout mice. *BMC Complement Altern Med.* 2015 Jul 15;15:232. PMID: 26174316 "The beneficial effects of *Illicium v.* [star anise] are consistent with a significant decrease in the iNOS-mediated inflammatory response, resulting in reduction of inflammation-associated gene expression. Treatment with *Illicium v.* may be the basis of a novel therapeutic strategy for hyperlipidemia-atherosclerosis."

Wu LD, Xiong CL et al. A new flavane acid from the fruits of *Illicium verum* [active against A549 lung cancer cells]. *Nat Prod Res.* 2016 Jan 6:1-6. PMID: 26734839 "Cytotoxicity evaluation of four compounds showed that illiciumflavane acid and (E)-1,2-bis(4-methoxyphenyl)ethene exhibited potential against A549 activities with IC50 values of 4.63 µM and 9.17 µM, respectively."

Stevia

Gregersen S, Jeppesen PB et al. Antihyperglycemic effects of stevioside [stevia extract] in type 2 diabetic subjects. *Metabolism.* 2004 Jan;53(1):73-6. PMID: 14681845. "Stevioside reduces postprandial blood glucose levels in type 2 diabetic patients, indicating beneficial effects on the glucose metabolism. Stevioside may be advantageous in the treatment of type 2 diabetes."

Misra H, Soni M et al. Antidiabetic activity of medium-polar extract from the leaves of Stevia rebaudiana Bert. (Bertoni) on alloxan-induced diabetic rats. *J Pharm Bioallied Sci.* 2011 Apr;3(2):242-8. PMID: 21687353. "Stevia extract was found to antagonize the necrotic action of alloxan and thus had a re-vitalizing effect on beta cells of pancreas."

Ozbayer C, Kurt H et al. Effects of Stevia rebaudiana (Bertoni) extract and N-nitro-L-arginine on renal function and ultrastructure of kidney cells in experimental type 2 Diabetes. *J Med Food.* 2011 Oct;14(10):1215-22. PMID: 21663490. "[Stevia]-treated diabetic rats had less mitochondrial swelling and vacuolization in thin kidney sections than other diabetic groups. ... Our results support the validity of [stevia] for the management of diabetes as well as diabetes-induced renal disorders."

Tamarind

Paula FS, Kabeya LM et al. Modulation of human neutrophil oxidative metabolism and degranulation by extract of *Tamarindus indica* L. fruit pulp. *Food Chem Toxicol.* 2009 Jan;47(1):163-70. PMID: 19022329. "The neutrophil reactive oxygen species generation, triggered by opsonized zymosan (OZ), n-formyl-methionyl-leucyl-phenylalanine (fMLP) or phorbol myristate acetate (PMA) ... was inhibited by ExT [tamarind extract] in a concentration-dependent manner. ExT was a more effective inhibitor of the PMA-stimulated neutrophil function ... than the OZ- ... or fMLP-stimulated cells. The ExT also inhibited neutrophil NADPH oxidase activity (evaluated by O_2 consumption), degranulation and elastase activity (evaluated by spectrophotometric methods) at concentrations higher than 200 microg/10(6)cells, without being toxic to the cells, under the conditions assessed."

World Health Organization. *Cough and Cold Remedies for the Treatment of Acute Respiratory Infection in Young Children.* 2001. WHO website: http://www.who. int/maternal_child_adolescent/documents/fch_cah_01_02/en/. "Antibiotic treatment, ... has no role in the management of children with the common cold because antibiotics do not shorten the duration of the illness and do not prevent complications or the development of pneumonia."

Tea (green or black)

Horiuchi Y, Toda M et al. Protective activity of tea and catechins against *Bordetella pertussis. Kansenshogaku Zasshi. 1992 May;66(5):599-605.* PMID: 1402092. "Green tea, black tea and coffee showed marked bactericidal activity [against *Bordetella pertussis*] at their concentrations in beverages."

Lee YL, Cesario T et al. Antibacterial activity of vegetables and juices. *Nutrition.* 2003 Nov-Dec;19(11-12):994-6. PMID: 14624951. "Tea also had significant activity, with bactericidal action in concentrations ranging up to 1.6 mg/mL, against a spectrum of pathogens including resistant strains such as methicillin- and ciprofloxacin-resistant staphylococci, vancomycin-resistant enterococci, and ciprofloxacin-resistant *Pseudomonas aeruginosa.*"

Matheson EM, Mainous AG 3rd et al. Tea and coffee consumption and MRSA nasal carriage. *Ann Fam Med.* 2011 Jul-Aug; 9(4): 299–304. PMID: 21747100. "In an adjusted logistic regression analysis controlling for age, race, sex, poverty-income ratio, current health status, hospitalization in the past 12 months, and use of antibiotics in the past month, individuals who reported consuming hot tea were one-half as likely to have MRSA nasal carriage relative to individuals who drank no hot tea (odds ratio = 0.47; 95% confidence interval, 0.31–0.71).”

Tea tree oil

Buck DS, Nidorf DM, Addino JG. Comparison of two topical preparations for the treatment of onychomycosis [toenail fungus]: Melaleuca alternifolia (tea tree) oil and clotrimazole [Lotrimin]. *J Fam Pract.* 1994 Jun;38(6):601-5. PMID: 8195735. “After 6 months of therapy, the two treatment groups were comparable based on culture cure (CL = 11%, TT = 18%) and clinical assessment documenting partial or full resolution (CL = 61%, TT = 60%). Three months later, about one half of each group reported continued improvement or resolution (CL = 55%; TT = 56%).”

Dryden MS, Dailly S, Crouch M. A randomized, controlled trial of tea tree topical preparations versus a standard topical regimen for the clearance of MRSA colonization. *J Hosp Infect.* 2004 Apr;56(4):283-6. PMID:15066738. “Tea tree treatment was more effective than chlorhexidine or silver sulfadiazine at clearing superficial skin sites and skin lesions. The tea tree preparations were effective, safe and well tolerated and could be considered in regimens for eradication of MRSA carriage.”

Tsao N, Kuo CF et al. Inhibition of group A streptococcal infection by Melaleuca alternifolia (tea tree) oil concentrate in the murine model. *J Appl Microbiol.* 2010 Mar;108(3):936-44. PMID: 1970933 “These results suggest that MAC [tea tree oil]may inhibit GAS [Group A Streptococcus]-induced skin damage and mouse death by directly inhibiting GAS growth and enhancing the bactericidal activity of macrophages. Our results provide scientific data on the use of MAC for the treatment of GAS-induced necrotizing fasciitis in the murine model.”

Vazquez JA, Zawawi AA. Efficacy of alcohol-based and alcohol-free melaleuca [tea tree oil] oral solution for the treatment of fluconazole-refractory oropharyngeal candidiasis in patients with AIDS. *HIV Clin Trials.* 2002 Sep-Oct;3(5):379-85. PMID: 12407487. “Both formulations of the melaleuca oral solution appear to be effective alternative regimens for patients with AIDS suffering from oropharyngeal candidiasis refractory to fluconazole.”

Thyme

Kemmerich B, Eberhardt R, Stammer H. Efficacy and tolerability of a fluid extract combination of thyme herb and ivy leaves and matched placebo in adults suffering from acute bronchitis with productive cough. A prospective, double-blind, placebo-controlled clinical trial. *Arzneimittelforschung.* 2006;56(9):652-60. PMID 17063641. “The symptoms of acute bronchitis (BSS) improved rapidly in both groups, but regression of symptoms was faster and the responder rates (p<0.0001) compared to placebo were higher at Visit 2 (83.0% vs 53.9%) and Visit 3 (96.2% vs. 74.7%) under the treatment of thyme-ivy combination.”

Tohidpour A, Sattari M et al. Antibacterial effect of essential oils from two medicinal plants against Methicillin-resistant Staphylococcus aureus (MRSA). *Phytomedicine.* 2010 Feb;17(2):142-5. PMID: 19576738. “Results revealed both [thyme and eucalyptus] oils to possess degrees of antibacterial activity against Gram (+) and Gram (-) bacteria. [Thyme essential oil] showed better inhibitory effects than [eucalyptus] oil.”

Turmeric *see* **Curcumin**

Valerian

Lindahl O, Lindwall L. Double blind study of a valerian preparation. *Pharmacol Biochem Behav.* 1989 Apr;32(4):1065-6. PMID: 2678162. "When compared with placebo [a preparation of just the sesquiterpene fraction of valerian] showed a good and significant effect on poor sleep (p less than 0.001). Forty-four percent reported perfect sleep and 89% reported improved sleep from the preparation. No side effects were observed."

Ziegler G, Ploch M et al. Efficacy and tolerability of valerian extract LI 156 compared with oxazepam in the treatment of non-organic insomnia—-a randomized, double-blind, comparative clinical study. *Eur J Med Res.* 2002 Nov 25;7(11):480-6. PMID: 12568976. "Most patients assessed their respective treatment as very good (82.8% in the valerian group, 73.4% in the oxazepam group). During the 6 week treatment phase Valerian extract LI 156 (Sedonium) 600 mg/die showed a comparable efficacy to 10 mg/die oxazepam [Serax, a benzodiazepine] in the therapy of non-organic insomnia."

Vitamin A

Elemraid MA, Mackenzie IJ et al. Nutritional factors in the pathogenesis of ear disease in children: a systematic review. *Ann Trop Paediatr.* 2009 Jun;29(2):85-99. PMID: 19460262. "Supplementation studies using single micronutrients and vitamins to determine efficacy in reducing acute or chronic otitis media provided some evidence for an association of middle-ear pathology with deficiencies of zinc or vitamin A."

Hakim F, Kerem E et al. Vitamins A and E and pulmonary exacerbations in patients with cystic fibrosis. *J Pediatr Gastroenterol Nutr.* 2007 Sep;45(3):347-53. PMID: 17873748 "Reduced serum levels of vitamin A and E even in the normal range are associated with an increased rate of pulmonary exacerbations in CF."

Karyadi E, West CE et al. A double-blind, placebo-controlled study of vitamin A and zinc supplementation in persons with tuberculosis [TB] in Indonesia: effects on clinical response and nutritional status. *Am J Clin Nutr.* 2002 Apr;75(4):720-7. PMID: 11916759 "Micronutrient deficiencies are common in patients with TB. ... Vitamin A and zinc supplementation improves the effect of TB medication after 2 mo of antituberculosis treatment and results in earlier sputum smear conversion."

Vitamin C

Biltagi MA, Baset AA et al. Omega-3 fatty acids, vitamin C and Zn supplementation in asthmatic children: a randomized self-controlled study. *Acta Paediatr.* 2009 Apr;98(4):737-42. PMID: 19154523. "There was a significant improvement of C-ACT, pulmonary function tests and sputum inflammatory markers with diet supplementation with omega-3 fatty acids, vitamin C and Zn (p < 0.001*)."

Jariwalla RJ, Roomi MW et al. Suppression of influenza A virus nuclear antigen production and neuraminidase activity by a nutrient mixture containing ascorbic acid, green tea extract and amino acids. Biofactors. 2007;31(1):1-15. PMID: 18806304. "The nutrient mixture exerts an antiviral effect against influenza A virus by lowering viral protein production in infected cells and diminishing viral enzymatic activity in cell-free particles."

McKeever TM, Scrivener S et al. Prospective study of diet and decline in lung function in a general population. *Am J Respir Crit Care Med.* 2002 May 1;165(9):1299-303. PMID: 11991883. "A high dietary intake of vitamin C, or of foods rich in this vitamin, may reduce the rate of loss of lung function in adults and thereby help to prevent chronic obstructive pulmonary disease."

Misso NLA, Petrovic N, et al. Plasma phospholipase A2 activity in patients with asthma: association with body mass index and cholesterol concentration. *Thorax.* 2008 Jan;63(1):21-6. PMID: 17573441. "Secretory phospholipases A2 (sPLA2) have functions relevant to asthmatic inflammation. ... Plasma vitamin C was inversely correlated with sPLA2 activity in patients with stable asthma and in control subjects."

Valenca SS, Bezerra FS et al. Supplementation with vitamins C and E improves mouse lung repair. *J Nutr Biochem.* 2008 Sep;19(9):604-11. PMID: 18155509 "These results indicate a possible role of vitamins C and E in lung repair after emphysema induced by long-term CS [cigarette smoke] exposure in mice."

Vitamin D

Clifford RL, Knox AJ. Vitamin D—a new treatment for airway remodelling in asthma? Br *J Pharmacol.* 2009 Nov;158(6):1426-8. PMID: 19906117. "Increased airway smooth muscle (ASM) mass plays a critical role in chronic asthmatic airway remodelling. ... This study identifies inhibition of ASM proliferation as a cellular effect of vitamin D and supports the hypothesis that vitamin D is a potential treatment for airway remodelling in asthma."

Ehlayel MS, Bener A, Sabbah A. Is high prevalence of vitamin D deficiency evidence for asthma and allergy risks? *Eur Ann Allergy Clin Immunol.* 2011 Jun;43(3):81-8. PMID: 21789969. "Serum vitamin D levels were lower in asthmatic than control. Vitamin D deficiency was higher among children with asthma, allergic rhinitis, atopic dermatitis, acute urticaria, and food allergy. In addition, [it] was associated with IgE atopy markers in asthmatic children more than controls."

Litonjua AA. Childhood asthma may be a consequence of vitamin D deficiency. *Curr Opin Allergy Clin Immunol.* 2009 Jun;9(3):202-7. PMID: 19365260. "Vitamin D may protect against wheezing illnesses through its role in upregulating antimicrobial proteins or through its multiple immune effects. In addition, vitamin D may play a therapeutic role in steroid resistant asthmatics, and lower vitamin D levels have recently been associated with higher risks for asthma exacerbations."

Zhao G, Ford ES et al. Low concentrations of serum 25-hydroxyvitamin D associated with increased risk for chronic bronchitis among US adults. *Br J Nutr* 2012 May;107(9):1386-92. PMID: 21899806. "For every 1ng/ml increase in 25(OH)D, the likelihood of having chronic bronchitis fell by 2.6% (P = 0.016)."

Vitamin E

Peh HY, Ho WE et al. Vitamin E isoform gamma-tocotrienol downregulates house dust mite-induced asthma. *J Immunol.* 2015 Jul 15;195(2):437-44. . PMID: 26041537. "Gamma-tocotrienol displayed better free radical-neutralizing activity in vitro and inhibition of BAL fluid total, eosinophil, and neutrophil counts in HDM mouse asthma in vivo, as compared with other vitamin E isoforms, including alpha-tocopherol. Besides, gamma-tocotrienol abated HDM-induced elevation of BAL fluid cytokine and chemokine levels, total reactive oxygen species and oxidative damage biomarker levels, and of serum IgE levels, but it promoted lung-endogenous antioxidant activities ... [It blocked] nuclear NF-kappaB level and enhance nuclear Nrf2 levels in lung lysates to greater extents than did ... prednisolone. It markedly suppressed methacholine-induced airway hyperresponsiveness in experimental asthma." Note the importance of using mixed-tocopherol, mixed-tocotrienol vitamin E, not the isolated alpha tocopherol commonly used in studies.

Wild Cherry Bark *(active ingredient benzoic acid)*

Armani E, Amari G et al. Novel class of benzoic acid ester derivatives as potent PDE4 inhibitors for inhaled administration in the treatment of respiratory diseases. *J Med Chem.* 2014 Feb 13;57(3):793-816. PMID: 24400806 "The first steps in the selection process of a new anti-inflammatory drug for the inhaled treatment of asthma and chronic obstructive pulmonary disease are herein described ... jn particular, esters of variously substituted benzoic acids were extensively explored, ... to maximize the inhibitory potency."

Yang MH, Kim J, et al. Nonsteroidal anti-inflammatory drug activated gene-1 (NAG-1) modulators from natural products as anti-cancer agents. *Life Sci.* 2014 Apr 1;100(2):75-84. PMID: 24530873 "Natural products are rich sources of gene modulators that may be useful in prevention and treatment of cancer [including] plant extracts belonging to ... *Prunus serotina* [wild cherry]."

Wild oats (Avena sativa)

Connor J, Connor T et al. The pharmacology of *Avena sativa* [wild oats]. *J Pharm Pharmacol.* 1975 Feb;27(2):92-8. PMID: 237083. "The pharmacology of *Avena sativa* has been investigated in laboratory animals following a report that tincture of *Avena sativa* reduced the craying for cigarettes in man. ...The pressor response to intravenously administered nicotine in urethane-anaesthetized rats was antagonized by prior administration of *Avena sativa*."

Xylitol

Bellanti JA, Nsouli TM. Xylitol Nasal Irrigation: A Possible Alternative Strategy for the Management of Chronic Rhinosinusitis. Oral Abstract #46. ACAAI Conference: 9 Nov. 2015. "In a study performed at Georgetown, researchers found that people who used a xylitol nasal spray had 35% higher peak air flow in the nose when compared to those who used saline alone."

Ferreira AS, Silva-Paes-Leme AF et al. Bypassing microbial resistance: xylitol controls microorganisms growth by means of its anti-adherence property. *Curr Pharm Biotechnol.* 2015;16(1):35-42. PMID: 25483720. "In this review, the effect of xylitol in inhibiting the growth of a different microorganism is described, focusing on studies in which such an anti-adherent property was highlighted."

Trahan L. Xylitol: a review of its action on mutans streptococci and dental plaque—its clinical significance. *Int Dent J. 1995* Feb;45(1 Suppl 1):77-92. PMID: 7607748 "When present in the oral environment xylitol not only prevents a shift of the bacterial community towards a more cariogenic microflora but also selects for a [*Streptococcus*] *mutans* population that was shown to have weakened virulence factors in preliminary in vitro experiments and in rats."

Weissman JD, Fernandez F, Hwang PH. Xylitol nasal irrigation in the management of chronic rhinosinusitis: a pilot study. *Laryngoscope.* 2011 Nov;121(11):2468-72. PMID: 21994147. "There was a significant reduction in SNOT-20 score during the xylitol phase of irrigation (mean drop of 2.43 points) as compared to the saline phase (mean increase of 3.93 points), indicating improved sinonasal symptoms (P = .0437). ... Xylitol in water is a well-tolerated agent for sinonasal irrigation. In the short term, xylitol irrigations result in greater improvement of symptoms of chronic rhinosinusitis as compared to saline irrigation."

Zabner J, Seiler MP et al. The osmolyte xylitol reduces the salt concentration of airway surface liquid and may enhance bacterial killing. *Proc Natl Acad Sci USA.* 2000 Oct 10;97(21):11614-9. PMID: 11027360. "Xylitol has a low transepithelial permeability, is poorly metabolized by several bacteria, and can lower the ASL salt concentration in both CF and non-CF airway epithelia in vitro. ... Xylitol sprayed for 4 days into each nostril of normal volunteers significantly decreased the number of nasal coagulase-negative Staphylococcus compared with saline control. "

Zinc

Brooks WA, Yunus M et al. Zinc for severe pneumonia in very young children: double-blind placebo-controlled trial. *Lancet.* 2004 May 22;363(9422):1683-8. PMID: 15158629. "Adjuvant treatment with 20 mg zinc per day accelerates recovery from severe pneumonia in children, and could help reduce antimicrobial resistance by decreasing multiple antibiotic exposures, and lessen complications and deaths where second line drugs are unavailable."

Meydani SN, Barnett JB et al. Serum zinc and pneumonia in nursing home elderly. *Am J Clin Nutr.* 2007 Oct;86(4):1167-73. PMID: 17921398. "Normal serum zinc concentrations in nursing home elderly are associated with a decreased incidence and duration of pneumonia, a decreased number of new antibiotic prescriptions, and a decrease in the days of antibiotic use. Zinc supplementation to maintain normal serum zinc concentrations in the elderly may help reduce the incidence of pneumonia and associated morbidity."

Mossad SB, Macknin ML et al., Zinc gluconate lozenges for treating the common cold: a randomized, placebo-controlled, double-blind study, *Annals in Internal Medicine,* 1996 Jul 15;125(2):81-88. PMID: 8678384 "The zinc group had significantly fewer days with coughing ... headache ... hoarseness ... nasal congestion... nasal drainage ... and sore throat [than the control group]."

Biltagi MA, Baset AA, et al. Omega-3 fatty acids, vitamin C and Zn supplementation in asthmatic children: a randomized self-controlled study. *Acta Paediatr.* 2009 Apr;98(4):737-42. PMID: 19154523. "There was a significant improvement of C-ACT, pulmonary function tests and sputum inflammatory markers with diet supplementation with omega-3 fatty acids, vitamin C and Zn (p < 0.001*)."

Summary of Specific
Homeopathic Medicines for Coughs

The chart appears on the next page.

If there is a *stress-related cause* or an *emotional shift* ...		
Emotion	Remedy	Other Distinguishing Symptoms
anxious about survival	Arsenicum	anxiety about money, job, home, security; restless after midnight
sudden fright	Aconite	scared to death such as a near-miss accident
humiliated	Aconite	spasmodic cough
hearing bad news	Ignatia	spasmodic cough
	Gelsemium	"droopy, drowsy, dizzy, dopy" like with the flu
grouchy	Bryonia	dry cough moving down into the chest; "leave me alone" painful cough, even pain of fractured ribs
separation	Pulsatilla	small children who cling to mom
sudden grief	Ignatia	spasmodic cough as if choking back sobs
long-term grief	Natrum mur.	egg white mucus
nervous tic	Cuprum	spasmodic cough, 3am, wants cold drinks

If you notice the *position they're in* when they cough...		
Position	Remedy	Other Distinguishing Symptoms
leaning forward	Kali carb.	lean elbows on knees; may wake coughing 2-4am
leaning over	Ipecac	vomit or feel like they might vomit up the mucus
lying down	Drosera	barking like a seal; one of the croup remedies

Dry Cough	
Bryonia	painful to cough, holds chest still; dry cough going down into chest
Phosphorus	cough from fumes. fragrances; dry cough going down into chest

Tickly Cough	
Rhus tox.	tickle in throat pit, may also have fever blisters
Rumex	tickle in the throat pit or at branching of trachea; from cold air

Croupy Cough	
Aconite	first stage of croupy cough, often waking at midnight
Drosera	barking like a seal, worse when lying down
Hepar sulph.	sensitive to hot and cold, to drafts, to being touched; irritable
Spongia	sounds like sawing wood

Productive (phlegmy, mucusy cough)	
Ant. Tart.	mucus deep in the chest; elderly and others too weak to get it up
Causticum	mucus around the larynx, can't get it up, stress incontinence
Hepar sulph.	soft yellow mucus rattling mid-chest; irritable, oversensitive
Kali bich.	thick, sticky, stringy mucus, hard to get out

ঌ APPENDIX F ঌ

Research Evidence for Homeopathy

Answering questions about homeopathy

When you use homeopathy you'll probably encounter questions from others—which is understandable, because it seems to defy common sense! (It does follow the laws of physics—a new branch called ultra high dilution physics—and we're getting to that.) I recommend waiting to tell anyone about your forays into homeopathy until you've had good results. Then to help you respond to questions, I'd like to present a conversation I had with my father, taken from my (Burke Lennihan's) previous book *Your Natural Medicine Cabinet.*

My father was a distinguished vascular surgeon who practiced medicine for nearly 60 years. He was enthusiastic about me but bewildered by my choice of profession. I grew up expecting to become a doctor like him or a research biochemist like my mother, who worked for Dr. Papanicolau, originator of the Pap smear.

My father the doctor helped me a lot in writing *Your Natural Medicine Cabinet* — by arguing with just about everything in it. "Where are the research studies?" he would say. "Show me the double-blind, randomized, placebo-controlled studies on this stuff and then I'll try it." So here's the deal, dad.

It would be ideal to have the National Institutes of Health give us money to research homeopathy, but in the meantime, I am recommending that readers listen to their bodies, try safe homeopathic remedies, notice what works, and trust their own experience. These natural medicines have 200 years of clinical experience to back up their safety and effectiveness.

"Let's take the case of smoking," I said — a topic dear to my father's heart. As a vascular surgeon (specializing in blood vessel surgery) he was a pioneer in recommending natural lifestyles. He would demand that his patients stop smoking, start exercising, and change to a low-fat diet, decades before these interventions became popular.

And he set a good example for his patients. He stopped smoking (he only smoked a pipe — ah, the aroma! — but he learned it could cause tongue and lip cancer). He started running marathons. He would get up at 4:30 in the morning so he could complete his marathon training and still get to the hospital by 7 am. If his patients told him they didn't have time to exercise, he brushed off the excuse. "If I have time, you have time," he would tell them.

"So dad, what if back in the 1960s, one of your colleagues told you he had noticed that his clients who stopped smoking had better circulation — based on their reports of fewer leg cramps, less shortness of breath while walking uphill, and no more cold hands and feet. Would you have started recommending right away that your patients stop smoking, knowing that they would get other benefits even if they weren't able to avoid surgery?

"Or, dad, would you refuse to recommend it until the research studies were completed, which could take 10 years? And what if no one would pay for the studies, since no industry would benefit from them? Would you go ahead and urge your patients to stop smoking anyway?"

"Sure," dad says. "Right away. No need to wait for the research."

"So it's the same with my stuff," I said. "It's harmless. It costs less than $10. It's likely to bring about other health benefits. There's no money for research studies. There are a lot of people telling us that it works for them. Like a little melt-in-your-mouth tablet that might help with those stomach cramps of yours."

"Okay," my 85-year-old surgeon-father says. "Let's give it a try."

The Vital Force: the body's healing energy

I tried to explain to my father one of homeopathy's central concepts, the Vital Force or the body's own self-healing mechanism. He thought about it for a while. "You know," he said, "let's take the example of two elderly ladies with venous ulcers" (the hard-to-heal ulcers in the legs of frail elderly people, one of his specialties as a vascular surgeon). "One lady is still married, lives near her grandchildren, is active in her church, and enjoys working in her garden. The other one is widowed, isolated, depressed, never goes out, never sees anyone. The first one will get better and the second one will not."

"That's it, dad!" I said. "The first lady has a strong Vital Force, that's why her body is able to heal. Did they teach you that concept in medical school?"

"No," my dad said, "but any doctor who's been in practice for a while is familiar with it." So the body's healing energy is *explicitly* addressed in the energy-based healing modalities like acupuncture and homeopathy, while it's a *silent* partner in mainstream Western medicine.

It's unproven, there's nothing in it—and it's dangerous?

I frequently hear two contradictory arguments against homeopathy: that there's nothing in it, and that it's dangerous. Neither of these assertions is true: homeopathic remedies do contain small amounts of the medicinal substance, as described on the next page, and a German study of more than 300 million doses of homeopathic remedies found only a few hundred reactions attributable to homeopathy.

Many critics say it's "unproven," which is also not true—there is extensive research supporting it—but in any case, remember that "unproven" does not mean "proven not to work." It means "not yet tested." In the case of homeopathy, that's due to a lack of funds and also to the *assumption* that it can't possibly be true, therefore not worth testing.

Homeopathy is said to work by the placebo effect, but that can't be true either, because double-blind trials have shown it to be effective on animals and small children. Veterinary homeopathy is well established, offering—among other things—safe, effective and inexpensive alternatives to antibiotics for farm animals. And parents who have given a remedy to a baby screaming with teething pain, and watched the child stop crying in their arms, know that it cannot possibly be the placebo effect.

Nor can the effect be based simply on a pleasant experience with a professional homeopath, as some claim. This was my father's theory. "You're a nice person and people like talking to you. That's why they feel better," he would say. No matter how supportive the experience, no matter how much the client enjoys feeling truly heard, that pleasant feeling won't last long and the remedy will not have a healing effect if it is not a good match.

The best proof of homeopathy's effectiveness is personal experience. Try the remedies in this book. Sometimes homeopathy does not work well for a particular person, but if you keep trying it on several people, you *will* see it work. Can it work for someone who doesn't "believe in it"? It can but in my experience these people tend to give up after one dose. ("See! This stuff doesn't work!") You wouldn't do that with a pharmaceutical! You may find it works most dramatically for your children and pets—and they'll be more compliant!

Research on homeopathy: it *does* exist

There is plenty of research, though most of it has been conducted overseas where homeopathy is an accepted part of the health care system. Dana Ullman, MPH has done such a thorough job of keeping track of this research and describing it, that I'll simply refer you to his Huffington Post blogs and to his website, www.homeopathic.com. His e-book, *Evidence-Based Homeopathic Family Medicine,* is worth getting because it documents the research for dozens of common complaints while providing more extensive remedy recommendations than I can give here. Ullman kindly allowed us to excerpt one of his research chapters later in this appendix. The book references more than 200 clinical studies that have been published in peer-reviewed medical journals, listed in the chapter for each condition.

A dramatic and compelling book about the science behind homeopathy is Dr. Amy Lansky's *Impossible Cure.* Lansky was a NASA computer scientist whose autistic son was cured with homeopathy (that's why it's called *Impossible Cure,* because conventional medicine considers autism incurable). She was so impressed that she left NASA to become a professional homeopath. Her book interweaves a report on the research documenting homeopathy with the compelling story of her son, who has now graduated from college.

A new development since Lansky's book: proof of homeopathy based on "outcomes" research, which means measuring the overall effectiveness of a modality. The Swiss government spent five years thoroughly examining the safety, effectiveness, and cost-effectiveness of homeopathy (with typical Swiss neutrality) and has decided to keep covering it in their national health insurance. The government study also reviewed all the available research on homeopathy and found the research on homeopathy for upper respiratory tract infections particularly compelling. The report itself is quite dry, but you don't need to wade through it because Dana Ullman has done an excellent job of summarizing it in his Huffington Post blog.

Homeopathy: the original nanopharmacology

Impossible Cure was also written before the new research on nanoparticles came out, and that's the most exciting new horizon in homeopathy research. Nanopharmacology is the latest development in conventional medicine—the discovery that tiny particles of a drug, just a few molecules wide, can be as effective as the full strength version while minimizing the side effects—and homeopathy was the original nanopharmacology. It's often said "homeopathy can't work because there's nothing in it," but it turns out that there *is* something in it: the original medicinal substance, in nanoparticle form. These particles are so tiny that they escaped detection until recently when they were scanned with a new technology called High Resolution Transmission Electron Microscopy.

Using this technique, the small particles of the remedy substance can be not only seen but also measured, and it turns out that the particles of the active ingredient are actually larger in high potency remedies. This makes sense in terms of how homeopathy works: we know from experience that higher potencies are more powerful. It makes no sense in terms of conventional chemistry and physics, because the higher potencies are more dilute, so there should be *less* of the starting substance.

But the effectiveness of homeopathy is based on the ways that water behaves *differently* when a substance is *highly* diluted in it, according to a new branch of physics called ultra high dilution physics. The latest research shows that water behaves differently when a substance has been highly diluted in it, *even after the substance is completely removed.*

The latest work of Nobel Laureate Dr. Luc Montagnier reveals that "DNA produces structural changes in water, which persist at very high dilutions, and which lead to resonant electromagnetic signals that we can measure," while distinguished Italian physicist Emilio del Giudice described these structural changes as "coherent domains ... resonating cavities produced by the electromagnetic field." That's more physics than my brain can handle, but the science wonks will find references for further study in the Endnotes.

How come my doctor says it's unproven?

Chances are your doctor is not familiar with the research on homeopathy, which is understandable, since it is not taught in American medical schools. Once they are in practice, physicians are busy keeping up with new developments in their own specialty, leaving little to no time for the new research emerging in other specialties like homeopathy.

Homeopathic drug manufacturers cannot afford to fund research the way American drug companies do. The U.S. government has funded a few studies that have demonstrated the effectiveness of homeopathy and have been published in peer-reviewed journals (such as one on homeopathy for childhood diarrhea, another for mild traumatic brain injury). Research on homeopathy for coughs is summarized in the rest of this appendix.

To reassure doctors, tell them that homeopathy is an accepted part of the national health care system in many countries around the world. The Swiss government has elevated homeopathy to the same status as conventional medicine, and in the US the FDA categorizes it as a form of over-the-counter medicine. Each homeopathic product has an NDC number (National Drug Code product identifier from the FDA) like other OTC medications.

Please be respectful and appreciative of all that doctors do know as you share your stories of success with homeopathy. Doctors will become more comfortable with natural healing the more they hear about their patients using it.

Research on homeopathy for coughs

Research on herbs and supplements for coughs is fairly self-explanatory, since these products are more amenable to conventional medical testing. Research on homeopathy requires more background information because homeopathy by its nature, with its **choice of remedy individualized to the patient**, is difficult to study with a randomized, placebo-controlled trial. What follows is the best explanation to date of research on homeopathy for coughs, extracted from Dana Ullman's e-book *Homeopathic Family Medicine* and reproduced here with his permission. Ullman is the leading expert on tracking research on homeopathy worldwide, and his e-book is the best single resource. Here's Dana:

Homeopathic medicines can help heal respiratory infections, though a persistent and/or extremely painful cough may require the attention of a professional homeopath. There have been several studies of patients with acute respiratory infection that have shown positive results with homeopathic treatment, and there was one very well conducted trial on people with chronic obstructive pulmonary disease with extremely positive results.

Books on physiology and pathology typically refer to the body's cough reflex as an important defensive function of the organism, and yet many conventional cough medicines are meant to suppress the cough. While such medicines provide temporary relief, they tend to prolong the ailment, and still worse, they tend to lead to various side effects that create their own problems.

The Swiss government commissioned a review of basic sciences and clinical trials testing homeopathic medicines (Bornhöft, Wolf, von Ammon, 2006). Their report noted 29 clinical studies in the domain 'Upper Respiratory Tract Infections/Allergic Reactions' showed a positive overall result in favor of homeopathy. They also found that in 6 out of 7 controlled studies, homeopathic medicines were at least equivalent to conventional medical interventions. They also found 8 out of 16 placebo-controlled studies were significant in favor of homeopathy.

In a randomized, double-blind, placebo-controlled trial, 80 patients with acute bronchitis were treated with either a homeopathic syrup or a placebo for a week (Zanasi, Mazzolini, Tursi, et al, 2013).

The composition of the homeopathic syrup was as follows:

Anemone pulsatilla 6 CH
Rumex crispus 6 CH
Bryonia dioica 3 CH
Ipecahuana 3 CH
Spongia tosta 3 CH
Sticta pulmonaria 3 CH
Antimonium tartaricum 6 CH
Myocarde 6 CH
Coccus cacti 3 CH
Drosera MT.

[Most of these remedies were described in chapter 5; the numbers following their names indicate the strength or potency – *Ed.*]

The subjects recorded cough severity in a diary by means of a verbal category-descriptive score for two weeks. Sputum viscosity was assessed with a viscosimeter before and after 4 days of treatment; patients were also asked to provide a subjective evaluation of viscosity. The 80 patients were randomized to receive placebo (n=40) or the homeopathic syrup (n=40). All patients completed the study.

In each group cough scores decreased over time, however, after 4 and 7 days of treatment, cough severity was significantly lower in the homeopathic group than in the placebo one ($P<0.001$ and $P=0.023$, respectively). Sputum was collected from 53 patients: in both groups its viscosity significantly decreased after 4 days of treatment ($P<0.001$); however, viscosity was significantly lower in the homeopathic group ($P=0.018$). However, the subjective evaluation did not significantly differ between the two groups ($P=0.059$). No adverse events related to any treatment were reported.

The researchers concluded that the homeopathic syrup employed in the study was able to effectively reduce cough severity and sputum viscosity, thereby representing a valid remedy for the management of acute cough induced by upper respiratory tract infections.

A randomized double-blind placebo controlled study of 175 children with recurrent respiratory infections was conducted at a university hospital (de Lange de Klerk, Bloomers, Kuik, et al, 1994). Children were prescribed an individually chosen homeopathic medicine or placebo. Those children given a homeopathic medicine showed 18% less daily symptoms than those given a placebo. The homeopathic group reduced their use of antibiotics by 55%, while the placebo group reduced their use by 38%. The homeopathic group also experienced 24% less adenoidectomies than the placebo group. Despite these seemingly impressive results, none reached statistical significance (the daily symptom score was P=.06).

An open, pragmatic, randomized parallel-group trial with waiting-list group as control was conducted in Norway (Steinsbekk, Fønnebø, Lewith, et al, 2005). One hundred and sixty-nine children below the age of 10 years, recruited by post from children previously diagnosed with URTI, were randomly assigned to receive either pragmatic homeopathic care from one of five homeopaths for 12 weeks or to a waiting-list control using self-selected, conventional health care.

There was a significant difference in median total symptom score in favor of homeopathic care (24 points) compared to the control group (44 points) (p = 0.026). The difference in the median number of days with URTI symptoms was statistically significant with 8 days in the homeopathic group and 13 days in the control group (p = 0.006). There was no statistical difference in the use of conventional medication or care between the two groups. Because of these results, the researchers concluded that there was a clinically relevant effect of individualised homeopathic care in the prevention of URTI in children.

A relatively small study of 30 children under 5 years of age who had been suffering from an upper respiratory tract infection was conducted (Ramchandani, 2010). This study compared the number of respiratory tract infections for the 6 months before treatment and the 6 months after treatment. This study utlized individually determined homeopathic treatment and was not blinded or randomized. The results showed a highly significant result in favor of homeopathic treatment. However, it is generally known that the older a child gets, the fewer respiratory tract infections s/he receives. Still, it seems that the difference between the before and after treatment suggests that homeopathic medicines may have had a beneficial effect, though no age-adjusted statistical analysis was provided.

The effectiveness of a homeopathic combination remedy, called Gripp-Heel, was compared with that of conventional treatments in a prospective, observational cohort study in 485 patients with mild viral infections and symptoms such as fever, headache, muscle pain, cough or sore throat (Rabe, Weiser, and Klein, 2004). Practitioners specialized in homeopathy or conventional treatment, or practiced both to similar extents. As evaluated by the practitioners, the homeopathic treatment was effective to similar or greater degree than the conventional therapies: 68% of patients were considered asymptomatic at the end of Gripp-Heel therapy vs. 48% of patients in the control group. Practitioners judged homeopathic treatments as 'successful' in 78% of cases vs. 52% for conventional therapies. Tolerability and compliance were good in both treatment groups, with the verdict 'very good' given for 89% of patients in the homoeopathic group vs. 39% in the conventional treatment group.

Ingredients of Gripp-Heel:

Aconitum napellus 4x 120 mg
Bryonia alba 4x
Lachesis mutus 12x 60 mg
Eupatorium perfoliatum 3x
Phosphorus 5x.

An open, multicenter, prospective, active-controlled cohort study in patients with inflammatory processes and diseases of the upper respiratory tract was conducted (Ammerschlager, Klein, Weiser, Oberbaum, 2005). Patients were given either Euphorbium compositum nasal drops (a Heel brand homeopathic formula product) or xylometazoline (Otrivine, a conventional decongestant drug), and the efficacy and tolerability was evaluated. This cohort study indicates a comparable efficacy and tolerability profile of the homeopathic complex remedy Euphorbium compositum nasal drops and the reference substance xylometazoline in patients with inflammatory processes and diseases of the upper respiratory tract. Non-inferiority of the homeopathic complex remedy to xylometazoline could be shown for all studied variables and in no case did the lower boundary of the 95% confidence interval cross the threshold of 0.5 score points.

One in vitro study tested a homeopathic formula product (Euphorbium compositum, by Heel) showed antiviral activity against respiratory syncytial virus (RSV) (Glatthaar-Saalmuller, 2001). Analyses of two of the three plant-derived ingredients of this formula (Euphorbium resomofera and Pulsatilla pratensis) reveal antiviral action against RSV. A minimal antiviral action against influenza A virus and human rhinovirus was also noted.

In addition to the above studies of primarily acute respiratory disease, there has been one important study of patients with more serious chronic respiratory disease.

A prospective, randomized, double-blind, placebo-controlled study with parallel assignment was performed to assess the influence of sublingually administered Kali bichromicum (potassium dichromate) 30C on the amount of tenacious, stringy tracheal secretions in critically ill patients with a history of tobacco use and COPD (chronic obstructive pulmonary disease) (Frass, Dielacher, Linkesch, et al, 2005). In this study, 50 patients received either Kali bichromicum 30C globules (group 1) or placebo (group 2). Five globules were administered twice daily at intervals of 12 hours. The amount of tracheal secretions on day 2 after the start of the study as well as the time for successful extubation and length of stay in the ICU were recorded.

The amount of tracheal secretions was reduced significantly in group 1 (p < 0.0001). Extubation could be performed significantly earlier in group 1 (i.e. they could breathe on their own without a mechanical ventilator, p < 0.0001). Similarly, length of stay was significantly shorter in group 1 (4.20 +/- 1.61 days vs 7.68 +/- 3.60 days, p < 0.0001 [mean +/- SD]). This data suggest that potentized (diluted and vigorously shaken) Kali bichromicum may help to decrease the amount of stringy tracheal secretions in COPD patients.

In this study, all patients underwent a trial of extubation, but none of the patients in group 1 had to be reintubated or needed even noninvasive ventilation to improve breathing. The amount of secretions remained stable and did not increase for patients in group 1. Also, the blood gas analyses after extubation remained stable in group 1. In contrast, four patients in group 2 had to be reintubated due to deterioration of blood gas analysis that was caused by tracheal secretions of grade 2 or 3.

Ammerschlager H, Klein P, Weiser M, Oberbaum M., Treatment of inflammatory diseases of the upper respiratory tract—comparison of a homeopathic complex remedy with xylometazoline [Article in German]. *Forsch Komplementarmed Klass Naturheilkd.* 2005 Feb;12(1):24-31.

Bornhöft G, von Ammon K, Maxion-Bergemann S, et al. Effectiveness, safety and cost-effectiveness of homeopathy in general practice—summarized health technology assessment. *Forsch Komplementmed.* 2006;13 Suppl 2:19-29.

de Lange de Klerk ESM, Blommers J, Kuik DJ, et al., Effect of homoeopathic medicines on daily burden of symptoms in children with recurrent upper respiratory tract infections, *BMJ*, November 19, 1994;309:1329-1332.

Frass M, Dielacher C, Linkesch M, et al. Influence of potassium dichromate on tracheal secretions in critically ill patients, *Chest,* March, 2005; 127:936-941.

Glatthaar-Saalmuller B, Fallier-Becker P. Antiviral action of Euphorbium compositum and its components. *Forsch Komplementarmed Klass Naturheilkd,* 2001;8:207-212.

Linde K, Clausius N, Ramirez G, et al., Are the clinical effects of homoeopathy placebo effects? a meta-analysis of placebo-controlled trials, *Lancet,* September 20, 1997, 350:834-843.

Rabe M. Weiser P. Klein, Effectiveness and tolerability of a homoeopathic remedy compared with conventional therapy for mild viral infections. *Int J Clin Pract.* 2004 Sep;58(9):827-32.

Ramchandani NM. Homoeopathic treatment of upper respiratory tract infections in children: Evaluation of thirty case series. *Complementary Therapies in Clinical Practice* 16 (2010):101-108.

Steinsbekk A, Fønnebø V, Lewith G, Bentzen N. a pragmatic, randomised, controlled trial comparing individualised homeopathic care and waiting-list controls. *Complementary Therapies in Medicine,* December 2005;13(4):231-238. PMID: 16338192.

Zanasi A, Mazzolini M, Tursi F, et al. Homeopathic medicine for acute cough in upper respiratory tract infections and acute bronchitis: a randomized, double-blind, placebo-controlled trial, *Pulmonary Pharmacology & Therapeutics* (2013), doi: 10.1016/j.pupt.2013.05.007. PMID: 23714686.

Research on Individual Homeopathic Remedies

Studies of individual homeopathic medicines are rarely conducted (and unlikely to be found effective) because homeopathy is based on treating each person with the homeopathic medicine most closely matching his/her symptoms. A specific chief complaint such as a cough can potentially be treated with several dozen remedies. This makes it difficult to isolate a particular remedy. Hence the use of combinations as in the last study below.

Arsenicum

Riveron-Garrotte M. *Ensayo clinico aleatorizado controlado del tratamento homeopatico de asma bronquial. Boletin Mexicano* 1998,31:54-61. Arsenicum was the second most frequently prescribed homeopathic medicine in this double-blind RCT in Cuba on patients with bronchial asthma. 97.4% improved and 87.2% reduced their use of conventional medicine vs. 12.5% improved and none reduced their meds in the placebo group.

Grindelia

Riveron-Garrotte M. *Ensayo clinico aleatorizado controlado del tratamento homeopatico de asma bronquial. Boletin Mexicano* 1998,31:54-61. Grindelia was the most frequently prescribed homeopathic medicine in this double-blind RCT in Cuba on patients with bronchial asthma. 97.4% improved and 87.2% reduced their use of conventional medicine vs. 12.5% improved and none reduced their meds in the placebo group.

Kali bichromicum [potassium dichromate]

Frass M, Dielacher C et al. Influence of potassium dichromate on tracheal secretions in critically ill patients. *Chest.* 2005 Mar;127(3):936-41. PMID: 15764779. "Extubation could be performed significantly earlier in group 1 [the Kali bichromicum group] (p < 0.0001, Table 2). Similarly, length of stay at the ICU was significantly shorter in group 1 (p < 0.0001, Table 2). [Kali bichromicum 30] may be able to minimize the amount of tracheal secretions and therefore to allow earlier extubation when compared to placebo ... due to a reduction in stringy, tenacious tracheal secretions."

Adler M. Efficacy and safety of a fixed-combination homeopathic therapy for sinusitis. *Adv Ther.* 1999 Mar-Apr;16(2):103-11. "At the first visit, after a mean of 4.1 days of treatment [with Sinusitis PMD, a combination of Lobaria pulmonaria, Luffa operculata and potassium dichromate], secretolysis had increased significantly and typical sinusitis symptoms, such as headache, pressure pain at nerve exit points, and irritating cough, were reduced."

Note that these studies used homeopathically diluted potassium bichromate. When used full strength it is extremely toxic.

For more information about homeopathy

My first book, *Your Natural Medicine Cabinet: A Practical Guide to Drug-Free Remedboses for Common Ailments,* was written to be the most user-friendly, empowering and accessible introduction to homeopathy.

Once you've mastered the simple concepts in my book, I recommend Dana Ullman's *Homeopathic Medicines for Children and Infants* and Dr. Dennis Chernin's *The Complete Homeopathic Resource Guide.*

Then when you are comfortable with the home prescribing guidelines in these books, you'll be ready for Miranda Castro's *Complete Homeopathy Handbook,* which will teach you homeopathy the way the pros do it but in a way that anyone can master it.

If you like learning the audiovisual way rather than from a book, you can view lively videos of Miranda, spiced with lots of stories and her British sense of humor, on Vimeo. Check my website, www.Green-HealingPress.com, for the link to the latest videos.

For healthcare professionals (and anyone interested in the research), the ideal book is Dana Ullman's *Evidence-Based Homeopathic Family Medicine.* It reviews the top remedies for each of more than 100 conditions, it provides an evaluation of all the available research for each one.

Research Evidence for Natural Therapies

Acupressure

Maa SH, Sun MF et al. Effect of acupuncture or acupressure on quality of life of patients with chronic obstructive asthma: a pilot study. *J Altern Complement Med.* 2003 Oct;9(5):659-70. PMID: 14629844. "Patients with clinically stable, chronic obstructive asthma experienced clinically significant improvements in quality of life when their standard care was supplemented with acupuncture or acupressure."

McFadden KL, Healy KM et al. Acupressure as a non-pharmacological intervention for traumatic brain injury (TBI). *J Neurotrauma.* 2011 Jan;28(1):21-34. Dec 27. PMID: 20979460. "These results suggest an enhancement in working memory function associated with active [acupressure] treatments."

Wu HS, Lin LC et al. The psychologic consequences of chronic dyspnea in chronic pulmonary obstruction disease: the effects of acupressure on depression. *J Altern Complement Med.* 2007 Mar;13(2):253-61. PMID: 17388769. "These findings provide health professionals with an evidence-based intervention to use with persons with COPD. Applying this acupressure program in clinical practice, communities, and long-term care units may lessen chronic dyspnea and depression in persons with COPD."

Breathing exercises

Slader CA, Reddel HK et al. Double blind randomised controlled trial of two different breathing techniques in the management of asthma. *Thorax.* 2006 Aug;61(8):651-6. PMID: 16517572 "[Use of short-acting beta(2) agonists] decreased by 86% (p<0.0001) and ICS [inhaled corticosteroid] dose was reduced by 50% (p<0.0001; p>0.10 between groups) [one group was taught shallow nasal breathing, the other group was taught upper body exercises]."

Thomas M. Are breathing exercises an effective strategy for people with asthma? *Nurs Times.* 2009 Mar 17-23;105(10):22-7. PMID: 19400340. "This study found that adult patients with asthma who were taught breathing exercises showed improvements in quality of life, symptoms and psychological well-being after six months. Breathing exercises may have a role in helping the many people treated for asthma in general practice who have symptoms despite inhaled treatment."

Buteyko breathing

Agency for Healthcare Research and Quality (US). http://www.effectivehealthcare. ahrq.gov Breathing Exercises and/or Retraining Techniques in the Treatment of Asthma: Comparative Effectiveness Review No. 71 (2012). The Buteyko breathing technique achieves "medium to large improvements in asthma symptoms and reductions in reliever medications" and "Available evidence suggests that selected intensive behavioural approaches that include breathing retraining exercises may improve asthma symptoms and reduce reliever medication use in motivated adults with poorly controlled asthma."

Cowie RL, Conley DP, et al. A randomised controlled trial of the Buteyko technique as an adjunct to conventional management of asthma. *Respir Med.* 2008 May;102(5):726-32. "Six months after completion of the interventions, a large majority of subjects in each group [one taught the Buteyko technique, the other taught breathing techniques by a physiotherapist] displayed control of their asthma with the additional benefit of reduction in inhaled corticosteroid use in the Buteyko group."

Austin G, Brown C et al. Buteyko breathing technique [BBT] reduces hyperventilation-induced hypocapnoea and dyspnoea after exercise in asthma. *Am J Respir Crit Care Med* 179;2009:A3409 "Our study demonstrated the hypothesised physiology of BBT ... By teaching patients to reduce hypernoea of breathing (the rate & depth), BBT may reduce asthma symptoms and improve exercise tolerance and control."

Opat AJ, Cohen MM et al. A clinical trial of the Buteyko Breathing Technique in asthma as taught by a video. *J Asthma* 2000;37(7):557-64. PMID: 11059522. "Our results demonstrated a significant improvement in quality of life among those assigned to the BBT compared with placebo (p= 0.043), as well as a significant reduction in inhaled bronchodilator intake (p = 0.008)."

Fasting

Fernandes G, Venkatraman JT, Turturro A, et al. Effect of food restriction on life span and immune functions in long-lived Fischer-344 x Brown Norway F1 rats. *J Clin Immunol* 1997 Jan; 17(1):17:85–95. PMID: 9049789. "These findings [with rats whose lifespan is 137 weeks on an ad libitum diet and 177 weeks on a food-restricted diet] indicate that food restriction may selectively act to maintain a lower number of antigen-induced memory T cells with age, thereby maintaining the organism's ability to produce higher levels of IL-2 with age. In summary, the increased cell-mediated immune function noted in aged FR rats appears to be due to the presence of a higher number of naive T cells, which are known to produce elevated levels of the antiinflammatory cytokines, which may in part be responsible for reducing the observed age-related rise in disease."

Heilbronn LK, de Jonge L, et al. Effect of 6-month calorie restriction on biomarkers of longevity, metabolic adaptation, and oxidative stress in overweight individuals:

a randomized controlled trial. *JAMA* 2006 Apr 5;295(13):1539-48. PMID: 16595757. "Our findings suggest that 2 biomarkers of longevity (fasting insulin level and body temperature) are decreased by prolonged calorie restriction in humans and support the theory that metabolic rate is reduced beyond the level expected from reduced metabolic body mass" [i.e. from the weight lost during six months of calorie restriction – Ed.].

Jolly CA. Dietary restriction and immune function. *J Nutr* 2004 134(8):1853-6. PMID:15284365. "Dietary restriction delays the onset of T-lymphocyte-dependent autoimmune disease; this may be attributed to improved antioxidant defense mechanisms. ... The beneficial effects of dietary restriction were shown in both the CD4 and CD8 T-lymphocyte subsets as well as in various immune compartments such as the spleen, mesenteric lymph nodes, peripheral blood, thymus, and salivary glands."

Nakamura S, Hisamura R et al. Fasting mitigates immediate hypersensitivity: a pivotal role of endogeous D-beta-hydroxybutyrate. *Nutrition & Metabolism* 2014 Aug. 28;11:40. PMID: 25302070. "Immediate hypersensitivity reaction was significantly suppressed by fasting. A significant reduction in mast cells degranulation... was observed in rat peritoneal mast cells delivered from the 24 hours fasting treatment."

Tovt-Korshyns'ka MI, Spivak MIa, Chopei IV. Short-term fasting therapy courses efficacy in preasthma and asthma patients. [article in Ukrainian] *Likars'ka Sprava* 2002;Apr-June;(3–4):79–81. PMID: 12145900. "In patients with preasthma and bronchial asthma, short-term courses of fasting dietotherapy (FDT) with a 7-day fasting period proved to be effective, as evidenced by clinical-and-functional and laboratory investigations. The incidence rate of viral infections was much lower with short-term courses compared to long-term courses. Short-term FDT courses with a 3-day fasting period have been found out to result in a significant decrease in the level of anxiety, as measured by Spilberger Anxiety Inventory."

Underwood DC, Matthews JK et al. Food restriction-mediated adrenal influences on antigen-induced bronchoconstriction and airway eosinophil influx in the guinea pig. *Int Arch Allergy Immunol* 1998 Sep;117(1):52-9. PMID: 9751848. " [after 18 hours of fasting] In addition to higher plasma levels of epinephrine (30% increase) and cortisol (33% increase), fasted guinea pigs had significantly lower (60% decreased) maximal bronchoconstrictor responses to OA than nonfasted, sensitized litter mates....We speculate that the reduced responsiveness to antigen in fasted versus fed animals may result from food-restriction-induced, stress-related release of epinephrine and cortisol from the adrenal glands, thereby suppressing mast cell degranulation or reducing responsiveness to spasmogenic and chemotactic mediators."

Yamamoto H, Suzuki J, Yamauchi Y: Psychophysiological study on fasting therapy. *Psychother Psychosom* 1979;32(1-4):229-240. PMID: 550177. "The peak [EEG] frequency decreased as fasting progressed, while it increased as re-fed continued. Percent energy of alpha waves after fasting therapy was significantly higher than that of the pre-fasting stage. ... It seems that ketone nutrition may work as a strong stressor in the brain cell, temporarily placing all biological mechanisms in a stress state and then activating the natural healing power inherent to the human body, thereby bringing about homeostasis."

Forest bathing

Li Q. Effect of forest bathing trips on human immune function *Environ Health Prev Med.*2010 Jan; 15(1): 9–17. PMID: 19568839 "Incorporating forest bathing trips ... has now become a recognized relaxation and/or stress management activity in Japan. The results of a study using the Profile of Mood States (POMS) test demonstrated that a forest bathing trip significantly increased the score for vigor and decreased the scores for anxiety, depression, and anger. Habitual forest bathing may help to decrease the risk of psychosocial stress-related diseases."

Li Q, Morimoto K et al. A forest bathing trip increases human natural killer activity and expression of anti-cancer proteins in female subjects. *J Biol Regul Homeost Agents.* 2008 Jan-Mar;22(1):45-55. PMID: 18394317. "The forest bathing trip significantly increased NK activity and the numbers of NK, perforin, granulysin, and granzymes A/B-expressing cells and significantly decreased the percentage of T cells, and the concentrations of adrenaline and noradrenaline in urine. The increased NK activity lasted for more than 7 days after the trip. ... Phytoncides released from trees and decreased stress hormone levels may partially contribute to the increased NK activity."

Gargles

Sakai M, Shimbo T et al. Cost-effectiveness of gargling for the prevention of upper respiratory tract infections. *BMC Health Serv Res.* 2008 Dec 16;8:258. PMID: 19087312. "This study suggests gargling as a cost-effective preventive strategy for URTI that is acceptable from perspectives of both the third-party payer and society."

Satomura K, Kitamura T et al. Prevention of upper respiratory tract infections by gargling: a randomized trial. *Am J Prev Med.* 2005 Nov;29(4):302-7. PMID: 16242593. "A Cox regression (proportional hazard model) revealed the efficacy of water gargling (hazard ratio=0.60, 95% CI=0.39-0.95). Even when a URTI occurred, water gargling tended to attenuate bronchial symptoms (p=0.055)."

Guided imagery

Menzies V, Taylor AG, Bourguignon C. Effects of guided imagery on outcomes of pain, functional status, and self-efficacy in persons diagnosed with fibromyalgia. *J Altern Complement Med.* 2006 Jan-Feb;12(1):23-30. PMID: 16494565. "This study demonstrated the effectiveness of guided imagery in improving functional status and sense of self-efficacy for managing pain and other symptoms of FM."

Menzies V, Kim S. Relaxation and guided imagery in Hispanic persons diagnosed with fibromyalgia: a pilot study. *Fam Community Health.* 2008 Jul-Sep;31(3):204-12. PMID: 18552601. "Visual imagery with relaxation is a mind-body intervention that may be used for symptom management in this population."

HEPA filters

Pedroletti C, Millinger E et al. Clinical effects of purified air administered to the breathing zone in allergic asthma: A double-blind randomized cross-over trial. *Respir Med.* 2009 Sep;103(9):1313-9. PMID: 19443189 "Clean air, administered directly to the breathing zone during sleep, can have a positive effect on bronchial inflammation and quality of life in patients with perennial allergic asthma."

van der Heide S, van Aalderen WM et al. Clinical effects of air cleaners in homes of asthmatic children sensitized to pet allergens. *J Allergy Clin Immunol.* 1999 Aug;104(2 Pt 1):447-51. PMID: 10452769. "In young asthmatic patients sensitized and exposed to pets in the home, application of [HEPA] air cleaners in living rooms and bedrooms was accompanied by a significant improvement in airway hyperresponsiveness and a decrease in peak flow amplitude."

Meditation

Barrett B, Hayney MS et al. Meditation or exercise for preventing acute respiratory infection: a randomized controlled trial. *Ann Fam Med.* 2012 Jul-Aug;10(4):337-46. PMID: 22778122. "Mean global severity was 144 for meditation, 248 for exercise, and 358 for control. ... There were 67 ARI-related days of-work missed in the control group, 32 in the exercise group (P = .041), and 16 in the meditation group (P <.001)."

Bower JE, Crosswell AD et al. Mindfulness meditation for younger breast cancer survivors: a randomized controlled trial. *Cancer.* 2015 Apr 15;121(8):1231-40. PMID: 25537522 "A brief, mindfulness-based intervention demonstrated preliminary short-term efficacy in reducing stress, behavioral symptoms, and proinflammatory signaling in younger breast cancer survivors."

Hoge EA, Chen MM et al. Loving-Kindness Meditation [LKM] practice associated with longer telomeres in women. *Brain Behav Immun.* 2013 Aug;32:159-63. PMID: 23602876. "Although limited by small sample size, these results offer the intriguing possibility that LKM practice [derived from Buddhism], especially in women, might alter RTL [relative telomere length], a biomarker associated with longevity."

Koike MK, Cardoso R. Meditation can produce beneficial effects to prevent cardiovascular disease. *Horm Mol Biol Clin Investig.* 2014 Jun;18(3):137-43. PMID: 25390009. "All types of meditation are associated with blood pressure control, enhancement in insulin resistance, reduction of lipid peroxidation and cellular senescence, independent of type of meditation. This review presents scientific evidence to explain how meditation can produce beneficial effects on the cardiovascular system."

Neti pots

Rabago D, Guerard E, Bukstein D. Nasal irrigation for chronic sinus symptoms in patients with allergic rhinitis, asthma, and nasal polyposis: a hypothesis generating study. *WMJ* 2008 Apr;107(2):69-75. PMID: 18593081 "Twelve of 21 subjects with allergic rhinitis spontaneously reported [in in-depth interviews] that HSNI [hypertonic saline nasal irrigation] improved symptoms. Two of 7 subjects with asthma and 1 of 2 subjects with nasal polyposis reported a positive association between HSNI use and asthma or nasal polyposis symptoms."

Prayer

Byrd RC. Positive therapeutic effects of intercessory prayer in a coronary care unit population. *South Med J.* 1988 Jul;81(7):826-9. PMID: 3393937. "The IP [intercessory prayer] group subsequently had a significantly lower severity score based on the hospital course after entry (P < .01). Multivariant analysis separated the groups on the basis of the outcome variables (P < .0001). The control patients required ventilatory assistance, antibiotics, and diuretics more frequently than patients in the IP group."

Cha KY, Wirth DP. Does prayer influence the success of in vitro fertilization-embryo transfer? Report of a masked, randomized trial. *J Reprod Med.* 2001 Sep;46(9):781-7. PMID:11584476. "The IP [intercessory prayer] group showed a higher [IVF] implantation rate (16.3% vs. 8%, P = .0005). Observed effects were independent of clinical or laboratory providers and clinical variables. ... A statistically significant difference was observed for the effect of IP on the outcome of IVF-ET, though the data should be interpreted as preliminary."

Lesniak KT. The effect of intercessory prayer [IP] on wound healing in nonhuman primates. *Altern Ther Health Med.* 2006 Nov-Dec;12(6):42-8. PMID: 17131981. "The [bush babies, small primates] were randomized to IP and L-tryptophan, or L-tryptophan only, for treatment of self-injurious behavior and related wounds. ... Prayer-group animals had a reduction in wound size compared to non-prayer animals (P=.028),... a greater increase in red blood cells (P=.006), hemoglobin (P=.01), and hematocrit (P=.018); a greater reduction in both mean corpuscular hemoglobin (P=.023) and corpuscular volume (P=.008); and a reduction in wound grooming (P=.01) and total grooming behaviors (P=.04) than non-prayer group animals. ... [Results] are consistent with prior human trials of IP effectiveness, but suggest IP-induced health improvements may be independent of confounds associated with human participants."

Matthews DA, Marlowe SM, MacNutt FS. Effects of intercessory prayer on patients with rheumatoid arthritis. *South Med J.* 2000 Dec;93(12):1177-86. PMID: 11142453. "Patients receiving in-person intercessory prayer showed significant overall improvement during 1-year follow-up. No additional effects from supplemental, distant intercessory prayer were found. ... In-person intercessory prayer may be a useful adjunct to standard medical care for certain patients with rheumatoid arthritis."

Saline nasal rinses

Pham V, Sykes K, Wei J. Long-term outcome of once daily nasal irrigation for the treatment of pediatric chronic rhinosinusitis. *Laryngoscope.* 2014 Apr;124(4):1000-7. PMID: 23712296 "Nasal irrigation is effective as a first-line treatment for pediatric chronic rhinosinusitis and subsequent nasal symptoms, and reduces the need for functional endoscopic sinus surgery and CT imaging."

Sowerby LJ, Wright ED. Tap water or "sterile" water for sinus irrigations: what are our patients using? *Int Forum Allergy Rhinol.* 2012 Jul-Aug;2(4):300-2. PMID: 22411733 "Patients almost uniformly reported improvement in their symptoms with the use of saline irrigations. ... However, tap water was used by 48% ... The extremely rare, but typically fatal, risk of meningoencephalitis ... makes this a potential health hazard."

Yoga

Khanam AA, Sachdeva U et al. Study of pulmonary and autonomic functions of asthma patients after yoga training. *Indian J Physiol Pharmacol.* 1996 Oct;40(4):318-24. PMID: 9055100 "The sympathetic reactivity was reduced following yoga training as indicated by significant (P < 0.01) reduction in DBP after HGT. The PIF (P < 0.01), BHT (P < 0.01) and CE (P < 0.01) showed significant improvement. The results closely indicated the reduction in sympathetic reactivity and improvement in the pulmonary ventilation by way of relaxation of voluntary inspiratory and expiratory muscles."

Nagarathna R, Nagendra HR. Yoga for bronchial asthma: a controlled study. *Br Med J (Clin Res Ed).* 1985 Oct 19;291(6502):1077-9. PMID: 3931802. "There was a significantly greater improvement in the group who practised yoga [including postures, pranayama and meditation] in the weekly number of attacks of asthma, scores for drug treatment, and peak flow rate."

Nagendra HR, Nagarathna R. An integrated approach of yoga therapy for bronchial asthma: a 3-54-month prospective study. *J Asthma.* 1986;23(3):123-37. PMID: 3745111. "The regular practitioners [of yoga postures, pranayama and meditation] showed the greatest improvement. Peak expiratory flow rate (PFR) values showed significant movement of patients toward normalcy after yoga, and 72, 69, and 66% of the patients have stopped or reduced parenteral, oral, and cortisone medication, respectively."

Singh S, Soni R et al. Effect of yoga practices on pulmonary function tests including transfer factor of lung for carbon monoxide (TLCO) in asthma patients. *Indian J Physiol Pharmacol.* 2012 Jan-Mar;56(1):63-8. PMID: 23029966. "[The group taught pranayama and yoga stretching] showed a statistically significant improvement (P<0.001) in Transfer factor of the lung for carbon monoxide (TLCO), forced vital capacity (FVC), forced expiratory volume in 1st sec (FEV1), peak expiratory flow rate (PEFR), maximum voluntary ventilation (MVV) and slow vital capacity (SVC) after yoga practice. Quality of life also increased significantly."

Sodhi C, Singh S, Dandona PK. A study of the effect of yoga training on pulmonary functions in patients with bronchial asthma. *Indian J Physiol Pharmacol.* 2009 Apr-Jun;53(2):169-74. PMID: 20112821. "[Subjects taught yoga breathing exercises] showed a statistically significant increasing trend (P < 0.01) in % predicted peak expiratory flow rate (PEFR), forced expiratory volume in the first second (FEV1), forced vital capacity (FVC), forced mid expiratory flow in 0.25-0.75 seconds (FEF25-75) and FEV1/FVC% ratio at 4 weeks and 8 weeks as compared to [the control group]."

Vedanthan PK, Kesavalu LN et al. Clinical study of yoga techniques in university students with asthma: a controlled study. *Allergy Asthma Proc.* 1998 Jan-Feb;19(1):3-9. PMID: 9532318. "The subjects in the yoga group [taught pranayama, yoga postures and meditation] reported a significant degree of relaxation, positive attitude, and better yoga exercise tolerance. There was also a tendency toward lesser usage of beta adrenergic inhalers."

❧ ENDNOTES ❧

Preface

i **France has the best health care in the world** "World Health Organization Assesses the World's Health Systems," http://www.who.int/whr/2000/media_centre/press_release/en/

i **95% of doctors in France prescribe homeopathy** Piolot M, Fagot JP et al. Homeopathy in France in 2011-2012 according to reimbursements in the French national health insurance database. *Fam Pract.* 2015 Aug;32(4):442-8. PMID: 25921648.

ii **Americans use natural healing** Eisenberg DM, Kessler FC et al. Unconventional medicine in the United States—prevalence, costs, and patterns of use. *N Engl J Med* 1993;328:246-252.
Tindle HA, Davis RB, Phillips RS, Eisenberg DM. Trends in use of complementary and alternative medicine by US adults: 1997-2002. *Altern Ther Health Med.* 2005 Jan-Feb;11(1):42-9. PMID: 15712765. In both studies, one-third of respondents used CAM in the previous year, representing about 72 million US adults.

Chapter One

6   St. Sauver JL, Warner DO et al. Why patients visit their doctors: assessing the most prevalent conditions in a defined American population. *Mayo Clin Proc.* 2013;88(1):56-67, PMID: 23274019. Upper respiratory conditions including asthma are the third most common category of diseases across the board among Americans living near the Mayo Clinic.

7   **most common cause of liver failure** "Acetaminophen poisoning [is implicated in] nearly 50% of all acute liver failure in this country [including] an estimated 458 deaths." Lee, WM. Acetaminophen and the US Acute Liver Failure Study Group: lowering the risks of hepatic failure. *Hepatology* 2004;40:6-9.

9   **Nelson Mandela quote**   From Mandela N, Hatang SK, Venter S. *Notes to the Future: Words of Wisdom.*

9   **C.S. Lewis quote**   from Lewis, C.S. *The Abolition of Man.*

Chapter Two

16   **government has asked doctors to stop prescribing antibiotics**   The "Get Smart" campaign of the CDC, FDA, American Academy of Pediatricians and others attempts to educate the public about the ineffectiveness of antibiotics for most colds, flus, coughs and other viral infections. "Key to combating antibiotic resistance is antibiotic stewardship, making sure we use the drugs appropriately—and only when needed." Sherman R, Cox E. Fighting antibiotic resistance. *FDA Voice* 11.14.12.

16   **President Obama's National Action Plan** for Combating Antibiotic Resistant Bacteria includes as its goals "identifying natural compounds with antibiotic activity (e.g., phytochemicals [and] essential oils." https://www.whitehouse.gov/sites/default/files/docs/national_action_plan_for_combating_antibotic-resistant_bacteria.pdf

18   **FDA review of over-the-counter medicines**   Any product that conforms to an OTC drug monograph (a kind of "recipe book" may be manufactured and sold without an individual product license. These monographs cover acceptable ingredients, doses, formulations, and labeling. They set the regulatory standard for the labeling and ingredients for products within a specific category such as antacids, analgesics, cough medications, etc. Finally, monographs are published in the government's Code of Federal Regulations (CFR) and the FDA's "stamp of approval" is placed on the label of any drug that conforms. However, the FDA doesn't thoroughly review these drugs the same way they review prescription medication.

21   **a homeopathic cough syrup compared to an antibiotic**   Zanasi A, Cazzato S et al. Does additional antimicrobial treatment have a better effect on URTI cough resolution than homeopathic symptomatic therapy alone? A real-life preliminary observational study in a pediatric population. *Multidiscip Respir Med.* 2015 Aug 7;10(1):25. PMID: 26251722, A homeopathic cough syrup plus an antibiotic was no more effective than the same syrup plus an antibiotic in children with a wet acute cough, in terms of the severity and duration of the cough, while the group with the antibiotic had more adverse effects (23% of the former group vs 5% of the homeopathy-only group).

In a somewhat comparable study of patients with upper respiratory tract infections, only half received a homeopathic medication while all had access to standard OTC medications for symptom relief, as needed. The homeopathy group's URIs resolved 1-2 days earlier even though they needed fewer OTC drugs and had fewer adverse events (3 of 265 patients in the homeopathy group compared to 8 of 258 in the OTC drugs-only group). Thinesse-Mallwitz M, Maydannik V et al. A homeopathic combination preparation in the treatment of feverish upper respiratory tract infections: an international randomized controlled trial. *Forsch Komplementmed.* 2015;22(3):163-70. PMID 26335189.

Chapter Three

29 **speed of cough droplets** Tang JW, Path FRC, Settles GS. Coughing and aerosols. *N Engl J Med* 2008; 359:e19October 9, 2008DOI: 10.1056/ NEJMicmo72576
Xie X, Li Y, et al. How far droplets can move in indoor environments—re-visiting the Wells evaporation-falling curve. *Indoor Air.* 2007 Jun;17(3):211-25.

30 **cough induced rib fractures** Hanak V, Hartman TE, Ryu JH. Cough-induced rib fractures. *Mayo Clin Proc* 2005 Jul;80(7):879-82. 54 patients at the Mayo Clinic had one or more fractured ribs from coughing over a nine-year period; women were more at risk, as were patients with osteopenia or osteoporosis.

Chapter Four

39 **aspirin from white willow bark** In the early 1800s a German chemist isolated an active ingredient and named it salicin (after Salix, the botanical name of the willow tree) and in 1899 the Bayer company synthesized a similar chemical, acetylsalicylic acid—or aspirin. This was the first time a chemical drug was created from a traditional plant medicine, and people have been using aspirin ever since. The German Commission E monographs (the international gold standard for herbal medicine) approve white willow bark for joint pain and occasional headaches. Hoffman, David. *Medical Herbalism* (2003) Healing Arts Press, p. 279.

39 **Andrew Weil "We forget about the plants."** Weil, Andrew. Why plants are (usually) better than drugs. Huffington Post, Nov. 19, 2010. http:// www.huffingtonpost.com/andrew-weil-md/why-plants-are-usually-be_b_ 785139.html

40 WHO, *Cough and Cold Remedies for the Treatment of Acute Respiratory Infections in Young Children.* Geneva, World Health Organization, 2001.

48 **cow's milk may affect mucus** Bartley J, McGlashan SR. Does milk increase mucus production? *Med Hypotheses.* 2010 Apr;74(4):732-4. PMID: 19932941. "Excessive milk consumption has a long association with increased respiratory tract mucus production and asthma," possibly explained by an exorphin breakdown product of A1 milk known to stimulate mucus production from gut mucus glands; the same substance in the blood could cause mucus secretion from respiratory glands.

41 **honey better than dextromethorphan** Paul IM, Beiler J et al. Effect of honey, dextromethorphan, and no treatment on nocturnal cough and sleep quality for coughing children and their parents. *Arch Pediatr Adolesc Med.* 2007 Dec ;161(12):1140-6. PMID: 18056558. "In a comparison of [buckwheat] honey, DM [dextromethorphan], and no treatment, parents rated honey most favorably for symptomatic relief of their child's nocturnal cough and sleep difficulty due to upper respiratory tract infection." *See page 207 for additional research on honey.*

45 **neti pots and saline rinses** See Appendix G, Research Evidence for Natural Therapies, for research studies on neti pots and saline rinses.

47 **research on vapor rubs** Paul IM, Beiler JS et al. Vapor rub, petrolatum, and no treatment for children with nocturnal cough and cold symptoms. *Pediatrics.* 2010 Dec;126(6):1092-9.

49 **chicken soup has immune activity** Rennard BO, Ertl RF, et al. Chicken soup inhibits neutrophil chemotaxis in vitro. *Chest.* 2000 Oct;118(4):1150-7.

50 **Fire Cider** Rosemary Gladstar's recipe from www.sagemountain.com used with permission.

Chapter Five *research on individual herbs and supplements in Appendix D*

53 **Neanderthal flower graves** Solecki R. *Shanidar: The First Flower People.* New York: Alfred A. Knopf, 1971.

65 **make your own custom-blended formula** see for example http://wellnessmama.com/3527/natural-vapor-rub/

65 **rosemary and lavender oil will not antidote homeopathic medicines** Miranda Castro, CCH, personal communication.

Chapter Six *research on homeopathy for coughs is in Appendix F*

82 **Kali bichromicum to thin tracheal secretions** Frass M, Dielacher C et

al. Influence of potassium dichromate on tracheal secretions in critically ill patients. *Chest.* 2005 Mar;127(3):936-41. PMID: 15764779. "Extubation could be performed significantly earlier in group 1 [the Kali bichromicum group] (p < 0.0001, Table 2). Similarly, length of stay at the ICU was significantly shorter in group 1 (p < 0.0001, Table 2). [Kali bichromicum 30] may be able to minimize the amount of tracheal secretions and therefore to allow earlier extubation when compared to placebo … due to a reduction in stringy, tenacious tracheal secretions."

88   **homeopathy works for animals**   As one example of the use of homeopathy in veterinary medicine:
Albrecht H, Schitte A. Homeopathy versus antibiotics in metaphylaxis of infectious diseases. *Alternative Therapies* 1999: 5(5), 64-68. Piglets crowded on a German livestock farm, highly susceptible to respiratory infections, were given either a homeopathic combination medicine, a subtherapeutic dose of antibiotics (the typical preventive dose), or placebo. The homeopathic formula successfully prevented URIs in the piglets, while the subtherapeutic dose was no more effective than placebo, calling into question the current practice of low-dose antibiotics used preventively.

88   **homeopathy works for small children**   Of the many research studies validating the use of homeopathy for small children, a series of three studies documented its effectiveness in childhood diarrhea, the top cause of death for small children worldwide.
Jacobs J, Jimenez LM, Gloyd SS. Treatment of acute childhood diarrhea with homeopathic medicine: a randomized double-blind controlled study in Nicaragua. *Pediatrics,* May, 1994,93,5:719-25. Half the children were given homeopathic medicine, half were given placebo, and all were given standard oral rehydration therapy. The combined results of this and two other studies using the same method showed a highly significant reduction in the duration of symptoms (P = 0.008). PMID: 8165068

89   **research on homeopathy**   The following recent research reviews address homeopathy in general.
Mathie RT et al. Randomised placebo-cotrolled trials of individualized homeopathic treatment: systematic review and meta-analysis. *Systematic Reviews,* 2014; 3:14.2. PMID: 25480654. This is the first study to look solely at placebo-controlled trials of individualized homeopathic treatment as delivered by homeopaths in practice. It is difficult to conduct a fair trial of homeopathy because the medicines are individualized and must be well

chosen by a professional homeopath. This review shows homeopathic medicines are 1.5 to 2 times more beneficial than placebo. The rigorous and transparent methodology, including a sensitivity analysis, gives credence to the findings.

Roberts R, Tournier A. The best studies show individualized homeopathic treatment has beneficial effects beyond placebo. *HRI Research Article 29:* Autumn 2015. In addition to reviewing the Mathie study just referenced, this article finds it more stringent in its criteria for reliability, included more up-to-date studies, and in other ways more sound than the previous meta-analyses by Shang, Ernst and others that failed to find benefit from homeopathy compared to placebo.

90   **nanopharmacology**   Chikramane PS, Suresh AK et al. Extreme homeopathic dilutions retain starting materials: A nanoparticulate perspective. *Homeopathy.* 2010 Oct;99(4):231-42. PMID: 20970092. "We have demonstrated for the first time by Transmission Electron Microscopy (TEM), electron diffraction and chemical analysis by Inductively Coupled Plasma-Atomic Emission Spectroscopy (ICP-AES), the presence of physical entities in these extreme dilutions [10^{60} and 10^{400}], in the form of nanoparticles of the starting metals and their aggregates."

91   **Montagnier's research on ultra high dilutions**   Montagnier L, Aissa J et al. Electromagnetic signals are produced by aqueous nanostructures derived from bacterial DNA sequences. *Interdiscip Sci Comput Life Sci* (2009) 1:81-90. http://www.ncbi.nlm.nih.gov/pubmed/20640822

91   **coherent domains**   Emilio del Giudice quoted in Ho, MW. *Living Rainbow H$_2$O.* Singapore: World Scientific and Imperial College Press, 2015.

91   **FDA categorizes homeopathy as OTC medications**   These regulations are based on the Homeopathic Pharmacopeia of the United States, www.hpus.com.

Chapter Seven

96   **Buteyko breathing**   see page 234 for research on the Buteyko method.

111   Jon Kabat-Zinn   Dr. Kabat-Zinn's books include *Mindfulness Meditation for Everyday Life, Mindfulness for Beginners,* and *Everyday Blessings: Mindfulness for Parents.* Research on his Mindfulness-Based Stress Reduction program is available at the website of the Center for Mindfulness at University of Massachusetts Medical School, www.umassmed.edu/cfm.

114   **Peggy Huddleston's work**   Huddleston, Peggy. *Prepare for Surgery, Heal Faster: A Guide of Mind-Body Techniques.* Cambridge, Mass.: Angel River

Press, 2012. Includes a CD of guided meditations. Research references are on the book's website, www.healfaster.com.

115 **Coué's affirmation** http://www.ukhypnosis.com/2009/06/17/emile-coues-method-of-%E2%80%9Cconscious-autosuggestion%E2%80%9D/

Chapter Eight

119 **not a single medical school offers a training course** see for example http://www.utsouthwestern.edu/education/medical-school/academics/curriculum/electives.html

125 **Dr. Richard Irwin,** chairman of the Cough Guidelines Committee of the American College of Chest Physicians and editor of the journal CHEST, in an NBC News interview, Jan. 9 2006

131 **Afrin causes rebound congestion** Graf P, Hallén H. One-week use of oxymetazoline nasal spray in patients with rhinitis medicamentosa one year after treatment. *ORL J Otorhinolaryngol Relat Spec.* 1997 Jan-Feb;59(1):39-44. PMID: 9104748 "[Patients] must be informed about the fast onset of rebound congestion upon repeated use in order to avoid the return of the vicious circle of nose drop abuse."

126 **longterm use of antihistamines can contribute to Alzheimer's** Gray SL, Anderson ML. Cumulative use of strong anticholinergics and incident dementia: a prospective cohort study. *JAMA Intern Med.* 2015 Mar;175(3):401-7. PMID: 25621434. "A 10-year cumulative dose-response relationship was observed for dementia and Alzheimer disease (test for trend, $P < .001$)."

Chapter Nine

139 **treating fever** Ray JJ, Schulman CI. Fever: suppress it or "let it ride"? *J Thorac Dis.* 2015 Dec;7(12):E633-6. PMID: 26793378. "The 'let it ride' philosophy has been supported by several recent randomized controlled trials."

149 **aspirin from white willow bark** In the early 1800s a German chemist isolated an active ingredient and named it salicin (after Salix, the botanical name of the willow tree) and in 1899 the Bayer company synthesized a similar chemical, acetylsalicylic acid—or aspirin. This was the first time a chemical drug was created from a traditional plant medicine, and people have been using aspirin ever since. The German Commission E monographs (the international gold standard for herbal medicine research) approve white willow bark for joint pain and occasional headaches. Hoffman, David. *Medical Herbalism* (2003) Healing Arts Press, p. 279.

149 **curcumin as good or better than ibuprofen**   Kuptniratsaikul V, Dajpratham P et al. Efficacy and safety of Curcuma domestica extract compared with ibuprofen in patients with knee osteoarthritis: a multicenter study. *Clin Interv Aging.* 2014;9:451-8. PMID: 24672232

149 **ibuprofen as dangerous as Vioxx**   Kelland K. High doses of common painkillers increase heart attack risks. Reuters 5/29/13. "Long-term high-dose use of painkillers such as ibuprofen or diclofenac is 'equally hazardous' in terms of heart attack risk as use of the drug Vioxx, which was withdrawn due to its potential dangers, researchers said on Thursday. Presenting the results of a large international study into a class of painkillers called non-steroidal anti-inflammatory drugs (NSAIDs), the researchers said high doses of them increase the risk of a major vascular event — a heart attack, stroke or dying from cardiovascular disease — by around a third."
Coxib and traditional NSAID Trialists' (CNT) Collaboration. Vascular and upper gastrointestinal effects of non-steroidal anti-inflammatory drugs: meta-analyses of individual participant data from randomised trials. *Lancet.* 2013 Aug 31;382(9894):769-79. PMID: 23726390. "Ibuprofen increased major coronary events ... but not major vascular events.... Heart failure risk was roughly doubled by all NSAIDs."

153 Gittleman, Ann Louise. *Zapped: Why Your Cell Phone Shouldn't Be Your Alarm Clock and 1,268 Ways to Outsmart the Hazards of Electronic Pollution.* HarperOne, 2012.

153 Dunckley, Victoria. *Reset Your Child's Brain: A Four-Week Plan to End Meltdowns, Raise Grades, and Boost Social Skills by Reversing the Effects of Electronic Screen-Time.* New World Library, 2015.

153 Adams, Case. *Natural Sleep Solutions for Insomnia: The Science of Sleep, Dreaming, and Nature's Sleep Remedies.* Logical Books, 2010.

Chapter Ten

159 **when doctors overprescribe antibiotics, resistance goes up**   Srinivasan A, associate director, CDC. Interview on PBS *Frontline,* June 28, 2013. http://www.pbs.org/wgbh/frontline/article/dr-arjun-srinivasan-weve-reached-the-end-of-antibiotics-period/

160 **recirculated air**   Zitter JN, Mazonson PD et al. Aircraft cabin air recirculation and symptoms of the common cold. 2002 Jul 24-31;288(4):483-6. In a study of over 1000 passengers flying from San Francisco to Denver, half were on planes with 50% recirculated air and the other half were on planes

with 100% fresh air. The subsequent rates of colds, runny noses and other upper respiratory symptoms were fundamentally the same in both groups. Leder K, Newman D. Respiratory infections during air travel. *Intern Med J.* 2005 Jan;35(1):50-5. "Studies of ventilation systems and patient outcomes indicate the spread of pathogens during flight occurs rarely." PMID: 15667469

162 **AAP says OTCs not effective for kids under six** https://www.aap.org/en-us/professional-resources/practice-support/pages/Withdrawal-of-Cold-Medicines-Addressing-Parent-Concerns.aspx. "Over-the-counter cough and cold medicines do not work for children younger than 6 years and in some cases may pose a health risk."

162 **research on the immune system of children in daycare** Coté SM, Petit-clerc A et al. Short- and long-term risk of infections as a function of group child care attendance: an 8-year population-based study. *Arch Pediatr Adolesc Med.* 2010 Dec;164(12):1132-7. PMID: 21135342

163 **landmark study** Gonzales R, Steiner JF, Sande MA. Antibiotic prescribing for adults with colds, upper respiratory tract infections, and bronchitis by ambulatory care physicians. *JAMA.* 1997 Sep 17;278(11):901-4. PMID: 9302241. "Although antibiotics have little or no benefit for colds, upper respiratory tract infections, or bronchitis, these conditions account for a sizable proportion of total antibiotic prescriptions for adults by office-based physicians in the United States. ... Therefore, effective strategies for changing prescribing behavior for these conditions will need to be broad based."

163 **antibiotics do not prevent pneumonia** WHO, *Cough and Cold Remedies for the Treatment of Acute Respiratory Infections in Young Children.* Geneva, World Health Organization, 2001.

Chapter Eleven

166 **Dr. Gus' interview on Z-Pak clinics** Painter K. Coughing for two weeks? You still don't need antibiotic. *USA Today* 1/14/13

168 **Cleveland Clinic article** Tofts RP, Ferrer G, Oliveira E. Q: How should one investigate a chronic cough? *Cleve Clin J Med.* 2011 Feb;78(2): 84-5, 89. PMID: 21285339

170 **incomplete history costs millions** Evidence Summary: Why focus on safety for patients with limited English proficiency? [US] Agency for Healthcare Research and Quality, professional education curriculum tool.

170 **medical errors cause more than 400,000 deaths per year** James JT.

A new, evidence-based estimate of patient harms associated with hospital care. *J Patient Safety.* Sept 2013;(9)3:122–128. PMID: 23860193 This review paper estimates from 210,000 to 400,000 deaths per year associated with preventable medical errors in hospital care, with serious harm to 10 to 20 times as many patients.

Deaths due to medical errors in outpatient settings may equal those in hospitals, according to a 2011 study, putting the combined total of deaths well into the hundreds of thousands. Bishop TF, Ryan AM, Casalino LP. Paid malpractice claims for adverse events in inpatient and outpatient settings. *JAMA.* 2011;305(23):2427-2431. PMID: 21673294.

170 **medical errors are the third leading cause of death** http://www.hospitalsafetyscore.org/newsroom/display/hospitalerrors-thirdleading-causeofdeathinus-improvementstooslow

171 **concerned with the overuse of X-rays** Braverman ER, Baker RJ, Loeffke B, Ferrer G. Combating radiation exposure before disaster strikes. *Townsend Letter for Doctors.* November 2012.

171 **overuse of X-rays well documented** Krishnan S. Radiation dose exceeds 50 mSv in 2% of ICU patients. Research presented at CHEST 2015, described in Zoler ML. Radiation dose exceeds 50 mSV [the US standard for safe annual workplace exposure] in 2% of ICU patients, in *CHEST Physician* online. One patient had radiation exposure more than four times the safe annual workplace limit. Dr. Krishnan suggests avoiding unnecessary radiation exposure to patients. http://www.chestphysician.org/specialty-focus/critical-care-medicine/article/radiation-exposure-exceeds-50-msv-in-2-of-icu-patients/f8f5bb0d1c3fb40a570cf3d6c56c9ac1.html

171 **ACE inhibitors can cause chronic cough** Research cited in Tofts RP, Ferrer G, Oliveira E. Q: How should one investigate a chronic cough? *Cleve Clin J Med.* 2011 Feb;78(2):84-5, 89. PMID: 21285339

177 **drugs that contribute to acid reflux by loosening the sphincter** from Harvard Health Publications, accessed via www.drugs.com

177 **stress increases the perception of acid reflux** Wright CE, Ebrecht M et al. The effect of psychological stress on symptom severity and perception in patients with gastro-oesophageal reflux. *J Psychosom Res.* 2005 Dec;59(6):415-24. PMID: 16310024. "The stressor induced a significant increase in cortisol and state anxiety; however, this was not associated with any increase in reflux... The perception of symptoms in the absence of increased reflux when one is stressed may account for low response rates to traditional treatments."

178 **acupuncture can help GERD**   Dickman R, Schiff E et al. Clinical trial: acupuncture vs. doubling the proton pump inhibitor dose in refractory heartburn. *Aliment Pharmacol Ther.* 2007;26(10):1333. 17875198. "Adding acupuncture is more effective than doubling the proton pump inhibitor dose in controlling [GERD]."

178 **PPIs interfere with vitamin and mineral absorption**   Heidelbaugh JJ. Proton pump inhibitors and risk of vitamin and mineral deficiency: evidence and clinical implications. *Ther Adv Drug Saf.* 2013 Jun; 4(3): 125–133 PMC4110863.

178 **risk of bone fractures**   In May 2010, the U.S. Food and Drug Administration (FDA) warned about the possible increased risk of fractures with PPI use. Information from studies suggests that PPIs may be associated with an increased risk of hip, wrist, and spine fractures. People who were at the greatest risk were those on high doses or used PPIs for at least one year or more. Source: PDRHealth.com. http://www.pdrhealth.com/proton-pump-inhibitors/side-effects-and-safety-of-proton-pump-inhibitors.

178 **dangerous lack of magnesium**   In March 2011, the FDA warned that using PPIs for more than a year may cause low magnesium levels. Symptoms of low magnesium include muscle spasms, tremors, irregular heartbeats, and seizures. Source: PDRHealth.com. http://www.pdrhealth.com/proton-pump-inhibitors/side-effects-and-safety-of-proton-pump-inhibitors.
Wang AK, Sharma S, Kim P, Mrejen-Shakin K. Hypomagnesemia in the intensive care unit: Choosing your gastrointestinal prophylaxis, a case report and review of the literature. *Indian J Crit Care Med.* 2014 Jul;18(7):456-60. doi: 10.4103/0972-5229.136075.
Cundy T, Dissanayake A. Severe hypomagnesaemia in long-term users of proton-pump inhibitors. *Clin Endocrinol (Oxf).* 2008 Aug;69(2):338-41. Epub 2008 Jan 23. PMID: 18221401

178 **prevent food-borne illnesses**   Bourne C, Charpiat B, et al. Emergent adverse effects of proton pump inhibitors. *Presse Med.* 2012 Dec 10. PMID: 23237784

178 **prevent Clostridium difficile**   Linsky A, Gupta K et al. Proton pump inhibitors and risk for recurrent Clostridium difficile infection. *Arch Intern Med.* 2010 May 10;170(9):772-8. PMID: 20458084
Freedberg DE, Lebwohl B, Abrams JA. The impact of proton pump inhibitors on the human gastrointestinal microbiome. *Clin Lab Med.* 2014

Dec;34(4):771-785. Epub 2014 Sep 24. PMID: 25439276

179 **prevent prion infection** Martinsen TC, Benestad SL, et al. Inhibitors of gastric acid secretion increase the risk of prion infection in mice. *Scand J Gastroenterol.* 2011 Sep 22. PMID: 21936725

179 **B$_{12}$ deficiency** Stomach acid is needed to release vitamin B$_{12}$ from the foods we eat. Because PPIs reduce stomach acid, it has been thought that PPIs may cause vitamin B$_{12}$ deficiency. Symptoms of vitamin B$_{12}$ deficiency may include weakness, anemia, numbness or tingling of hands or feet, memory problems, poor balance, and soreness of the tongue or mouth, according to the Physician's Desk Reference.

179 **inhibit effectiveness of vitamin C** Henry EB, Carswell Ca, et al. Proton pump inhibitors reduce the bioavailability of dietary vitamin C. *Aliment Pharmacol Ther.* 2005 Sep 15;22(6):539-45. PMID: 16167970

179 **rebound acid can be worse** Reimer C, Søndergaard B, et al. Proton-pump inhibitor therapy induces acid-related symptoms in healthy volunteers after withdrawal of therapy. *Gastroenterology.* 2009 Jul;137(1):80-7, 87.e1. PMID: 19362552

179 **take a capsule of betaine hydrochloride** This can work as well as a protein pump inhibitor to resolve symptoms of GERD, based on clinical experience. In a research study, it worked as well when combined with other supplements:
Pereira, R de S. Regression of gastroesophageal reflux disease symptoms using dietary supplementation with melatonin, vitamins and amino acids: comparison with omeprazole. *J Pineal Res.* 2006 Oct;41(3):195-200. PMID: 16948779. A supplement containing melatonin, vitamins B6 and B12, l-tryptophan, l-methionine and betaine hydrochloride provided complete regression of GERD symptoms (with no side effects) compared to only 65% of the control group on omeprazole.

179 **a glass of water can have the same effect** Karamanolis G, Theofanidou I, et al. A glass of water immediately increases gastric pH in healthy subjects. *Dig Dis Sci.* 2008 Dec;53(12):3128-32. PMID: 18473176

179 **orange peel extract for acid reflux** Sun, J. D-limonene [active ingredient in orange peel]: safety and clinical applications. *Alt Med Rev* 12(3);2007:259-264. By day 14, 86% of participants in one small study and 89% of those in another achieved complete relief of symptoms compared to 29% in the control group.

181 **Gutsy Chewy** Brown R, Sam CH et al. Effect of [Gutsy Chewy's pro-

prietary blend] on subjective ratings of gastro esophageal reflux following a refluxogenic meal. *J Diet Suppl.* 2015 Jun;12(2):138-45. PMID: 25144853. "[With a] proprietary blend of licorice extract, papain, and apple cider vinegar ... adjusted mean ± SEM heartburn score (15-min postmeal to 240 min) was significantly lower ... mean acid reflux score was significantly lower ... than in placebo treatment (0.72 ± 0.19 vs. 1.46 ± 0.19 cm; p = 0.013)."

180 **floating "raft" of an algae derivative**   research on Gaviscon, the commercial version, has demonstrated that the algae "raft" keeps stomach acid in the stomach; however Gaviscon is not recommended because it also contains aluminum hydroxide, and aluminum salts are implicated in Alzheimer's.

Rohof WO, Bennink RJ et al. An alginate-antacid formulation localizes to the acid pocket to reduce acid reflux in patients with gastroesophageal reflux disease. *Clin Gastroenterol Hepatol.* 2013 Dec;11(12):1585-91. "The alginate-antacid raft localizes to the postprandial acid pocket and displaces it below the diaphragm to reduce postprandial acid reflux."

Walton JR. Chronic aluminum intake causes Alzheimer's disease: applying Sir Austin Bradford Hill's causality criteria. *J Alzheimers Dis.* 2014;40(4):765-838. "AD [Alzheimer's disease] is a human form of chronic aluminum neurotoxicity. The causality analysis demonstrates that chronic aluminum intake causes AD." PMID: 24577474.

180 **training the diaphragm to contract the sphincter**   Eherer AJ, Netolitzky F et al. Positive effect of abdominal breathing exercise on gastroesophageal reflux disease: a randomized, controlled study. *Am J Gastroenterol.* 2012 Mar;107(3):372-8. PMID: 22146488. "We show that actively training the diaphragm by breathing exercise can improve GERD as assessed by pH-metry, QoL scores and PPI usage."

Chapter Twelve

186 **stop smoking with natural therapies**   see also Appendix G for additional research on the effectiveness of acupuncture, hypnosis, massage, mindfulness meditation and physical activity.

186 **stop smoking with acupuncture**   He D, Medbø JI, Høstmark AT. Effect of acupuncture on smoking cessation or reduction: an 8-month and 5-year follow-up study. *Prev Med.* 2001 Nov;33(5):364-72. "This study confirms that adequate acupuncture treatment may help motivated smokers

to reduce their smoking, or even quit smoking completely, and the effect may last for at least 5 years. Acupuncture may affect the subjects' smoking by reducing their taste of tobacco and their desire to smoke."

186 **stop smoking with hypnosis**   Carmody TP, Duncan C et al. Hypnosis for smoking cessation: a randomized trial. *Nicotine Tob Res.* 2008 May;10(5):811-8. PMID: 18569754

Green JP, Lynn SJ. Hypnosis and suggestion-based approaches to smoking cessation: an examination of the evidence. *Int J Clin Exp Hypn.* 2000 Apr;48(2):195-224. PMID: 10769984

186 **stop smoking with hand or ear massage**   Hernandez-Reif M, Field T, Hart S. Smoking cravings are reduced by self-massage [on hands or ears]. *Prev Med.* 1999 Jan;28(1):28-32. PMID: 9973585

186 **stop smoking with mindfulness meditation**   Bowen S, Marlatt A. Surfing the urge: brief mindfulness-based intervention for college student smokers. *Psychol Addict Behav.* 2009 Dec;23(4):666-71. PMID: 20025372

186 **stop smoking with physical activity**   Daniel J, Cropley M et al.. Acute effects of a short bout of moderate versus light intensity exercise versus inactivity on tobacco withdrawal symptoms in sedentary smokers. *Psychopharmacology* (Berl). 2004 Jul;174(3):320-6. PMID: 14997270

Prochaska JJ, Sharon M Hall SM et al. Physical activity as a strategy for maintaining tobacco abstinence: a randomized trial. *Prev Med.* 2008 Aug;47(2):215-20. PMID: 18572233

186 **stop smoking with herbs**   Mattioli L, Perfumi M. Evaluation of *Rhodiola rosea* L. extract on affective and physical signs of nicotine withdrawal in mice. *Swed Dent J.* 2006;30(2):55-60. PMID:19939867

Catania MA, Firenzuoli F et al. *Hypericum perforatum* attenuates nicotine withdrawal signs in mice. *Psychopharmacology* (Berl). 2003 Sep;169(2):186-9. PMID: 12719964

Ruedeberg C, Wiesmann UN et al. (St John's wort) extract Ze 117 inhibits dopamine re-uptake in rat striatal brain slices. An implication for use in smoking cessation treatment? *Phytother Res.* 2009 Jul 7. PMID: 19585471

187 **black pepper**   Rose JE, Behm FM. Inhalation of vapor from black pepper extract reduces smoking withdrawal symptoms. *Drug Alcohol Depend.* 1994 Feb;34(3):225-9. PMID: 8033760. "Reported craving for cigarettes was significantly reduced in the pepper condition relative to each of the two control conditions. In addition, negative affect and somatic symptoms of anxiety were alleviated in the pepper condition relative to the unflavored

placebo." *Black pepper extract also protects against lung cancer: see Appendix D.*

189 **yoga routine for COPD**   Presentation at CHEST 2015 by Dr. Randeep Guleria, described at CHEST Physician online (includes a video of Dr. Guleria discussing the study): http:/www.chestphysician.org/?id=33765 &tx_ttnews[tt_news]=447241&cHash=5335ee73a3c3a5468aa67565f27f325.

189 **xylitol**   Many research studies have shown that xylitol (a natural sweetener) reduces bacteria in the upper respiratory tract and in the mouth, where it prevents cavities. For example: Trahan L. Xylitol: a review of its action on mutans streptococci and dental plaque--its clinical significance. *Subst Abuse Treat Prev Policy.* 2008 Jan 25;3:1. PMID: 7607748 "When present in the oral environment xylitol not only prevents a shift of the bacterial community towards a more cariogenic microflora but also selects for a [Streptococcus] mutants population that was shown to have weakened virulence factors in preliminary in vitro experiments and in rats."

189 **EarthSweet** also contains chicory extract (Cicohorium intiba) as a source of fructooligosaccharides, substances that nourish the "garden" of healthy microbes in the gut, plus they improve digestion, increase bowel regularity, and fat metabolism; pretty much the opposite effect of white sugar.

Chapter Thirteen

193 **many unproven controversial treatments in Western medicine**
Dossey L, Chopra D, Roy R. The mythology of science-based medicine. Huffington Post, 11/7/2011. "The *British Medical Journal* recently undertook an general analysis of common medical treatments to determine which are supported by sufficient reliable evidence. They evaluated around 2,500 treatments, and the results were as follows:
46 percent of medical treatments were unknown in their effectiveness.
13 percent were found to be beneficial
23 percent were likely to be beneficial
Eight percent were as likely to be harmful as beneficial
Six percent were unlikely to be beneficial
Four percent were likely to be harmful or ineffective ...
This is remarkably similar to the results Dr. Brian Berman found in his analysis of completed Cochrane reviews of conventional medical practices. There, 38 percent of treatments were positive and 62 percent were negative or showed 'no evidence of effect.' "

Appendix C

200 **Americans spent \$40 billion on OTC drugs** Consumer Healthcare Products Association website. www.chpa.org/OTCvalue.aspx. Accessed February 15, 2015.

200 **\$7.7 billion on drugs for respiratory issues** IRI. www.iriworldwide. com. 2015.

202 **greater motivation for employees to participate in lifestyle changes** Williams-Piehota PA, Sirois FM et al. Agents of change: how do complementary and alternative medicine [CAM} providers play a role in health behavior change? *Altern Ther Health Med.* 2011 Jan-Feb;17(1):22-30. PMID: 21614941. "[CAM] provider support, increased responsibility for one's health, and the CAM treatments themselves contribute to behavior change." The principle reasons patients reported making such changes included the [CAM] treatment *made them feel well enough* to make the health behavior changes (53%), feeling better due to treatment *acted as a motivator* to change behavior (53%), ... and treatments themselves helped (48%).

202 **reduced employee turnover costs** Thornton, L. (2013). *Whole Person Caring: An interprofessional model for healing and wellness.* Indianapolis, IN: Sigma Theta Tau International Honor Society of Nursing. Cited in Oberg E, Guarneri M, Herman P, Walsh T. *Integrative Health and Medicine: Today's Answer to Affordable Healthcare.* Integrative Healthcare Policy Consortium, published online, available at http://www.ihpc.org/wp-content/uploads/IHPC-CE-Booklet-March2015.pdf "The implementation of Whole-Person Caring programs emphasizing self-care, self-healing practices and lifestyle changes among hospital employees significantly decreased turnover, reducing costs by \$1.5 million per year. In addition, patient satisfaction significantly improved (even through the program didn't treat patients directly)."

203 **Therapeutic Order** http://www.ndhealthfacts.org/wiki/Therapeutic_Order

203 **Initiative for Healthcare Improvement's Triple Aim** http://www.ihi.org/ engage/initiatives/tripleaim/Pages/default.aspx

203 **National Strategy for Quality Improvement in Health Care, 2011** http://www.ahrq.gov/workingforquality/reports/annual-reports/nqs2011 annlrpt.htm

203 **Dr. Berwick brings the Triple Aim to CMS** http://healthaffairs.org/ blog/2010/09/14/berwick-brings-the-triple-aim-to-cms/

203 **CAM saved \$367 a year** Lind BK, Lafferty WE, et al. Comparison of

health care expenditures among insured users and nonusers of complementary and alternative medicine in Washington State: a cost minimization analysis. *J Altern Complement Med.* 2010 Apr;16(4):411-7. PMID: 20423210.

203 Saputo, Len and Ben Belitsos. *A Return to Healing: Radical Health Care Reform and the Future of Medicine.* San Rafael, CA: Origin Press, 2009. Duggan, Robert. *Breaking the Iron Triangle: Reducing Health-care Costs in Corporate America.* Columbia, MD: Wisdom Well Press, 2012.

Appendix F

230 **Swiss government** www.swissinfo.ch.eng/complementary-therapies-swiss-to- recognise-homeopathy-as-legitimate-medicine/42053830

✷ ACKNOWLEDGEMENTS ✸

This journey of writing a book has given the term "team work" a whole new meaning. Books begin with an idea and are completed by the organized efforts of a team. I have been blessed with the help of many. I want to stop, take a deep breath, fill my lungs and hopefully without coughing say: Thank you!

First, to Dr. Michael Roizen of the Cleveland Clinic, who inspired me to write books and communicate health awareness. His encouragement ignited the flame of creativity in me, and I will be forever grateful.

Miranda Castro, CCH, for introducing me to Burke, and for her contributions to the chapter on homeopathy and the section on fevers.

U.S. Army Major General (Ret) Bernard Loeffke, who went on to become a physician's assistant and missionary after his retirement. I admire him as a fountain of knowledge. His contributions, advice and comments are much appreciated.

Dr. William Jana and his wife Wendy, for their guidance and for the blessing of meeting them.

Lisa Tener, the best book coach one can ever dream to have, for editing, helping us to organize our ideas, and putting us in touch with great like-minded people.

Liz Neporent, master writer and media expert whose knowledge has helped me navigate this new field of endeavor.

Our medical team: Dr. Ramirez, Roxana Karimzadeh, Fanny Tse, Tara Rowland, Jamellah Abraham, Alice Raff, Aliza Aronin, and John Way.

Dr. Elena Rios, President and CEO of the National Hispanic Medical Association, for her leadership and support.

The Cleveland Clinic Florida Team, especially my nurse Darlene Iglesias, the best nurse ever and cofounder of the Cleveland Clinic Cough Clinic.

Dr. Kaiser G. Lim of Mayo Clinic Rochester, for allowing me the privilege of learning from his cough center.

Dr. Smolley and Dr. Oliveira for supporting the Cough Clinic idea.

Professor Dr. Jose Muñiz, for being a great teacher; together with his wife Ana Maria, for being a model of integrity.

The wonderful nurses at the Cleveland Clinic ICU for offering a special kind of medicine, the one that combines knowledge and compassion.

Dr. Bill Kernan, Director of Pharmacy Services and Residency Program Director, for his help and guidance when the book was just an idea.

Jared West, Lic. Ac., for his contributions to the acupressure protocols and the Cleveland Clinic Ohio Wellness Center.

Dr. Marlow Hernandez and his team for their friendship and support during my time of transition.

Dr. Lisa Corsa for her support and for providing tough love to my patients, taking them to the next level with her expert physical therapy.

Dr. Antonio Briceño for his friendship and his contribution in translating this book into Spanish.

Peter Miret for being a moral compass in business leadership.

The nurses and respiratory therapists at Kindred of Hollywood Florida for opening their hearts to our team and embracing compassion daily.

Dr. Arlene Grant for kindling the fire of this campaign.

Craig Hoover, Dr. Carlos Corrales, and Ivan Vallejo, for their friendship, support and guidance.

My Pulmonary Fellowship buddies: Dr. Hector Yuseff Vazquez Saad, Dr. Salvador Villason, Dr. Hazam Ubasissi, Jeff Williams and Dr. Jalil Ahari, thanks for making my fellowship a memorable one.

My beloved patients from whom I continue to glean wisdom and knowledge, especially Ana Maria Garcia for her radiant attitude despite any circumstance. Jack (Zaydeh) and Iris (Bubbeh) for adopting my family and showering us with love. Wanda Nutt for your generous heart. Beba and Rin who take me back to my Cuban roots.

JD Rivera for his contagious faith. His prayers and nuggets of spiritual guidance are a powerhouse and they have greatly impacted me. Doris and Helio Munoz for always being there for me. Jose Barlart for his valuable support.

To all who have helped mold me to into who I am today: my mentors in Cuba, Dr. Edilberto Gonzalez Ochoa, Dr. Salvador Vidal Reve, Dr. Fidel Creach, Dr. Elejaldel, Enrique Riguiferos, Dr. Jacobus De Waard. The United Nations University team in Venezuela: Dr. Armando Mesa and Dr. Manny Rivera. Distinguished professor Dr. Guillermo Gutierrez and the staff of the

George Washington University Pulmonary and Critical Care team, just to name a few.

The best office team I can ever dream to have: Samantha Feola, my Operational Manager, for taking a leap of faith, for her support and "fabulous" attitude. Jayson Escalona, my Multi Media Manager for using his God-given talents to develop a concept into a masterpiece. Loren Pizarro for her support and amazing winning attitude. Ally Furey, for her sweet and peaceful demeanor. Luis Cairo, for his willingness and determination to make a difference.

My parents Miguelina (Grandma Lina) and Domingo (Grandpa Guito) for giving me life and the best family on the planet.

My brother Yoel and sister-in-law Bertha. Although they came in at the tail end of the book writing, they have been a tremendous help. They are the depiction of a servant's heart.

My wonderful sister-in-law Yami Schneider for her continued prayers.

My mother-in-law Alicia "Abby" for her willingness to help.

To the love of my life Nicole, for the countless hours you put into this journey with me. I couldn't have done it without you. I'm convinced God opened the floodgates of heaven and blessed me the day I met you. You inspire me every day.

My beloved children from whom I learn something new daily. Diego's desire to change the world encourages me, Amanda's compassion and tenderness inspires me, and Lauren's optimism and determination motivates me. I am honored to be called your Daddy.

Above all I want to thank my Lord Jesus Christ for rescuing me.

—*Gustavo Ferrer, MD*

I would like to thank my mother, Marjory Reynolds Lennihan, who inspired me with a love of native plants, which she uses in her wildflower gardens and I use as natural medicines. I would also like to thank my father, vascular surgeon Richard Lennihan, MD. I still feel his enthusiasm and encouragement for my life work in natural healing, even though he is no longer with us here on earth. Both of my parents infused in me a love of reading, of nature, of helping people, of making the world a better place, which I hope shines through in this book.

My advisers and helpers, without whom this book would not be possible:

Michelle Dossett, MD, PhD, MPH of Massachusetts General Hospital for her information on stress and acid reflux.

June Riedlinger Shibley, ND, PharmD, founder of the former Center for Integrative Therapy in Pharmaceutical Care at Massachusetts College of Pharmacy and Health Sciences and now supervising one of its clerkship rotations in integrative medicine; and her PharmD students, as well as Dr. John D. Coleman, for helping to research our recommendations.

Dana Ullman for sharing his compendium of research on homeopathy.

Jerry Kantor, LicAc, CCH, MMHS of Vital Force Health Care in Needham, Mass. and Teaching Associate at Harvard Medical School, for his assistance with the acupressure points for coughs.

Hadas Golan, MS CCC-SLP for information on Buteyko breathing.

Ann Z. Bauer, ScD, for sharing her doctoral dissertation "Developmental Effects of Analgesics: State of the Epidemiologic Evidence" with invaluable information about the harmful effects of acetaminophen.

Adam Stark of Debra's Natural Gourmet, Concord, Mass. and Elizabeth Stagl, CNS, of Cambridge Naturals, Cambridge, Mass., for advising me on the best current supplements.

Alycia Metz, for polishing the book with her proofreading.

My clients who shared their stories and our advance readers who gave us valuable feedback. Thank you all.

I know I speak for Dr. Gus when I say that we cannot take any credit for this book. We feel blessed to be the instruments of a higher power whom we call God or the Supreme Being. Coming from different approaches to medicine as well as different faith traditions, we hope to help defuse polarization, "reach across the aisle" and find common ground among all who seek better forms of healing. We respect others with different views and different sources of inspiration. As one of the great Doctors of the Church put it,

Omne verum, a quocumque dicatur, a Spiritu Sancto est. *

"All truth, by whomever it is spoken, is from the Holy Spirit."

We end this journey where we began: with spirit, with breath, and with gratitude for the inspiration that created this book.

—*Burke Lennihan, RN, CCH*

---

*St. Thomas Aquinas, quoting one of the early Church Fathers. Translation by Prof. Ralph Lazzaro, former Director of Language Studies at Harvard Divinity School.

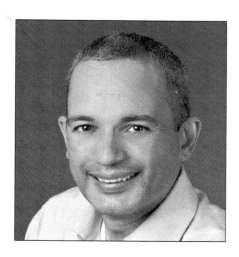

Dr. Gustavo Ferrer's life encompasses both traditional and modern forms of medicine. He grew up in a remote rural area of Cuba where health care consisted of his grandmother's herbal teas; and as Director of Respiratory Research for the U.N. in Venezuela, he witnessed the healing methods of one of the oldest tribes in South America. He was trained as a physician and pulmonologist in Cuba. In 2000 he came to the US and retrained with a residency in Texas and a pulmonary and critical care fellowship at George Washington University in DC. He then joined the Cleveland Clinic Florida where he founded the Cough Center. He has delivered over 100 presentations at local, national, and international medical meetings and is currently involved in multiple research studies.

In 2011, Dr. Ferrer was appointed to the prestigious National Steering Committee for the COPD Alliance of nine medical organizations, representing the National Hispanic Medical Association. As part of this esteemed group, he attended a White House briefing to discuss the Affordable Care Act. He has since received several prestigious awards, including: Best Doctors in the US by *U.S. News & World Report,* Most Compassionate Doctor, Patients' Choice Award, and multiple teaching awards.

Dr. Ferrer has been featured in *USA Today,* NBC News, CNN en Español, the *Miami Herald,* and on Radio Caracol Miami. He was also featured in many Latin American national newspapers. He is continually striving to improve healthcare in America, and in 2013 Gustavo Ferrer founded Intensive Care Experts Pulmonary Network. He can be reached at:

www.GustavoFerrerMD.com.

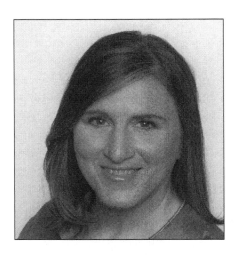

Burke Lennihan RN, CCH (Certified Classical Homeopath) has spent over 30 years in different aspects of holistic health care. She currently practices homeopathy at the Lydian Center for Innovative Health-care in Cambridge, Mass. and is the author of *Your Natural Medicine Cabinet: A Practical Guide to Drug-Free Remedies for Common Ailment*s.

After graduating from Harvard University at the top of her class, she operated health food stores in Boston and Cambridge for 16 years, where she developed her expertise in natural remedies. In 1996 she cofounded and administered the Renaissance Institute of Classical Homeopathy with her mentor, internationally distinguished homeo-path Dr. Luc De Schepper. She subsequently directed Teleosis School of Homeopathy from 2002 to 2009.

A visiting lecturer at Massachusetts College of Pharmacy and Health Sciences, Burke coauthored the homeopathy chapter in the American Pharmacists Association's *Handbook of Non-Prescription Drugs*. With more than 35 years of experience in meditation, she teaches classes in heart-center meditation at Harvard University's Center for Wellness and has lectured on holistic health there and at Lesley University.

Burke has taught physicians about homeopathy at the Integrative Medicine residency of Tufts University School of Medicine and at the Integrative Medicine for Underserved Populations conference.

She can be reached at www.YourNaturalMedicineCabinet.com.

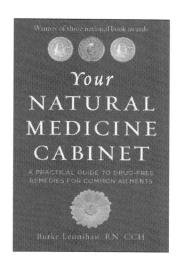

Also by Burke Lennihan

Your NATURAL MEDICINE CABINET

A Practical Guide to Drug-free Remedies for Common Ailments

winner of three
national book awards

In an engaging, entertaining style, *Your Natural Medicine Cabinet* makes it easy to find the latest information on healing over 100 common ailments with natural products. Ideal for families, busy households, and anyone interested in natural alternatives for themselves and their children, it offers essential resources in a concise, user-friendly format.

This easy-to-understand guide covers everything from acid reflux, flu, and insomnia to earaches, constipation, hemorrhoids, and thinning hair.

It introduces a new concept — emotional first aid, providing safe and effective natural treatments to use instead of pharmaceuticals — and it includes extensive information about homeopathic medicines, the best-kept secret in the natural pharmacy.

"This treasure trove of practical remedies is so well-written and understandable that it will appeal to a wide audience. Lennihan's years of experience and her knowledge of the literature that evaluates holistic approaches makes this a perfect addition to one's home library."
— Judy Norsigian, bestselling author of *Our Bodies, Ourselves*

"What bursts with common sense, vital information and is a comfort to have nearby? The answer is Burke Lennihan's splendid reference, *Your Natural Medicine Cabinet*. Cheerfully crammed with practical tidbits of natural healing lore, *Your Natural Medicine Cabinet* belongs in every home."
—Jerry Kantor, LicAc, CCH, Director, Vital Force Health Care
    Teaching Associate, Harvard Medical School

Single copies available online, $15
Multiple copies at a discount from
www.YourNaturalMedicineCabinet.com

Made in the USA
Lexington, KY
08 February 2019